Recent Research in Psychology

WITHDRAWN
UTSA LIBRARIES

Oliver Chadwick H. Ross Anderson
J. Martin Bland John Ramsey

Solvent Abuse
A Population-Based
Neuropsychological Study

Springer-Verlag
New York Berlin Heidelberg London Paris
Tokyo Hong Kong Barcelona Budapest

Oliver Chadwick
MRC Child Psychiatry Unit
Institute of Psychiatry
De Crespigny Park
London SE5 8AF
United Kingdom

H. Ross Anderson
Department of Public Health Sciences
St. George's Hospital Medical School
Cranmer Terrace
London SW17 0RE
United Kingdom

J. Martin Bland
Department of Medical Statistics
St. George's Hospital Medical School
Cranmer Terrace
London SW17 0RE
United Kingdom

John Ramsey
Department of Chemical Pathology
Toxicology Unit
St. George's Hospital Medical School
Cranmer Terrace
London SW17 0RE
United Kingdom

With two figures.

Library of Congress Cataloging-in-Publication Data
Solvent abuse: a population-based neuropsychological study / Oliver Chadwick . . . [et al.].
    p.   cm. — (Recent research in psychology)
    Includes bibliographical references and index.
    ISBN 0-387-97607-8 (alk. paper). — ISBN 3-540-97607-8 (alk. paper)
    1. Solvent abuse — Complications and sequelae.
2. Neuropsychological tests. I. Chadwick, Oliver. II. Series.
[DNLM: 1. Neuropsychology. 2. Solvents. 3. Substance Abuse-psychology.   WM 270 N494]
RC568.S64N48   1991
616.86 — dc20
DNLM/DLC
for Library of Congress   91-4871

Printed on acid-free paper.

Camera-ready copy provided by the authors.
Printed and bound by BookCrafters, Inc., Chelsea, MI.
Printed in the United States of America.

9 8 7 6 5 4 3 2 1

ISBN 0-387-97607-8 Springer-Verlag New York Berlin Heidelberg
ISBN 3-540-97607-8 Springer-Verlag Berlin Heidelberg New York

Acknowledgments

The study described in this book was carried out at St George's Hospital Medical School and we acknowledge with gratitude the help we received from others at different stages of the research. In particular, we would like to thank Corrine Moy, Clare Byrne, Stephen Bailey, Simon Walker and Andrew Tickle who helped with the collection and analysis of the data, Professor Andrew Mathews who offered constructive advice during the early stages of the research, Jaymala Solanki who typed the manuscript and the Audio Visual Services Department of St George's Hospital Medical School who transformed it into camara-ready form.

Our thanks are due to the staff at each of the participating schools for allowing us to conduct the study and for helping in a variety of ways. Virtually all of the information collected during the course of the study came directly from the pupils themselves and we are grateful to them for completing the questionnaires and for consenting to be interviewed and tested.

The study was supported by a grant from the British Government Department of Health and Social Security. It should go without saying however that the views expressed in the report are those of the authors and not necessarily those of the Department.

Contents

1 Introduction

1.1 History of Solvent Abuse

The practice of deliberately inhaling various gases or vapors in order to induce an altered state of mood or sensibility is not new. As noted repeatedly in other reviews (eg, Cohen, 1973; Novak, 1980), it was recognized in early Greek civilization as an adjunct to divination; indeed, it has now become customary, if not obligatory, to refer to the Oracle at Delphi before considering the more recent history of the subject. According to legend, the priestess at the Temple at Delphi would achieve communion with the Gods by inhaling the naturally-occurring gas that emanated from a fissure in a rock. Inhalation would induce a trance-like state. Her mystical observations and utterances while in this state were interpreted by the Temple Prophet and issued as divine pronouncements to those seeking guidance.

Incenses, perfumes and spices have probably always been used in ceremonial worship and religious ritual. However, in sofar as it is possible to make the distinction, these substances have been used primarily for their aromatic qualities rather than for their intoxicating effects.

The recreational use of gases and vapors dates from the end of the eighteenth century and may be seen as a concomitant of the scientific advances that preceded the industrial revolution. Following the synthesis of nitrous oxide by   Sir Joseph Priestley in 1776, the potential uses of the gas were explored in depth by Sir Humphrey Davy. According to Nagle (1968), Davy's discovery in 1799 of the anaesthetic properties of nitrous oxide was preceded by extensive informal experimentation in which he and his colleagues investigated its euphoriant properties on themselves and each other. The recreational use of the gas soon became popular among the well-connected and "genteel" and Coleridge, Southey, Roget and Sir Josiah Wedgewood were among those who tried this latest product of the Enlightenment.

Ether and chloroform also enjoyed popularity during the nineteenth century and 'ether frolics' became a fashionable form of entertainment particularly among medical students in Britain and the United States. Baudelaire and de Maupassant were among those who are said to have found inspiration in ether (Preble and Laury, 1967). However, its widespread popularity in Ireland following massive efforts to curb the use of alcohol soon began to cause concern. Towards the end of the century, under pressure from the temperance societies and faced with the loss of tax revenues, the problem was considered by a British parliamentary committee. Legislation to limit the sale of ether was subsequently introduced, but it was probably not until the 1920s, when alcohol became more readily available that the practice died out (Nagle, 1968).

Reports of petrol sniffing among rural adolescents in the USA began to appear in the early 1950s (eg, Clinger and Johnson, 1951; Faucett and Jensen, 1952), and following reports of glue sniffing among teenagers arrested in Colorado and elsewhere in the western United States the practice rapidly became epidemic (Brecher, 1974). Whether the practice actually started in the west and then spread eastward, as claimed by a number of commentators, is not entirely clear, but certainly the publicization of glue sniffing as a new and extraordinary teenage fad seems to have followed this route. Sporadic reports of solvent abuse in other parts of the world began to appear at about the same time. Nylander (1962), for example, reporting an epidemic of thinners abuse in Sweden wrote as follows:

"For about 10 years it has been employed in Sweden . . as an intoxicant, especially by older children and adolescents. This abuse of thinner, known as "sniffing", occurred in about 1955 literally as an epidemic in certain parts of Stockholm and the larger towns. It was reported that at times the abuse was widespread in the schools; and "sniffing" took place even during lessons . . . . . Subsequently the abuse of thinner decreased, but it is still used . . . . . by children and adolescents, and every year a number of cases of prolonged and severe abuse are admitted to the psychiatric clinics." (Nylander, 1962).

It is uncertain when sniffing first became popular among adolescents in the United Kingdom. Single case reports of petrol and glue sniffing first appeared during the early 1960s (eg, Oldham, 1961; Merry and Zachariadis, 1962; Bethell, 1965), but it was probably not until the beginning of the next decade that the practice began to achieve popularity (Watson, 1986). During the second half of the 1970s, the practice rapidly became more widespread (Watson, 1986) and the number of fatalities attributable to solvent abuse throughout the country showed a marked increase (Anderson, Macnair and Ramsey, 1985).

The range of readily available products that have been abused is wide. In addition to petrol, thinners and the various solvent-based glues, the list includes paints, lacquers, varnishes, aerosol products, dry cleaning and degreasing agents, nail varnish and more recently typewriter correction fluids and butane gas. As new products have become available, their recreational potential has been quickly discovered and exploited. One exception to this rule is amyl nitrite which was initially used for relief from angina in the nineteenth century but which became popular as a recreational substance only during the 1960s and 1970s when it was unofficially marketed for its reputed aphrodisiac (vasodilating) qualities.

1.2 The Abused Substances

Table 1 lists some of the more frequently abused products together with the main volatile components they contain. Some products may have a range of possible constituents or contain mixtures, but those shown in the table may be regarded as typical. The list includes the various cements and plastic glues, fuel gases such as butane, dry-cleaning and degreasing agents, typewriter correction fluids, anaesthetic agents and aerosols. Some are flammable. Unannounced changes are occasionally made in the chemical composition of some branded products and consequently reports describing the abuse of particular *chemicals* may be incorrect unless chemical analysis has actually been carried out.

It is important to appreciate that these volatile substances vary in their physical as well as in their chemical properties. In particular, they vary greatly in their boiling points, some being gases and others being liquids at room temperature. Table 2 lists the compounds found in the products listed in Table 1 with their boiling points and occupational exposure limits. Cardiac toxicity in animals appears to be related to boiling point (Clark and Tinston, 1982), the higher the boiling point the greater the risk. Toxicity is increased by prior sensitisation by adrenergic stimulation. The lower boiling compounds however carry a greater risk of exposure to very high concentrations due to their less controlled methods of administration. The occupational exposure limit permits comparison of the toxicity of different volatile substances in industrial settings.

On inhalation, the substances pass rapidly into the blood from the alveoli. They are very lipophilic (ie, are preferentially absorbed into fatty organs such as fat stores and brain). They are subsequently slowly excreted either unchanged through the lungs or as metabolites in urine. Some, such as toluene, may be detected as long as 10 days after the last exposure.

The acute risk of death associated with the abuse of various products depends partly on the concentration of the vapour that is inhaled, and this in turn depends on the method of abuse as well as on the proportion of very volatile components in the product. Products containing a high proportion of volatile components (eg, aerosols or butane) are likely to result in more concentrated vapours. Also, methods to facilitate the inhalation of very concentrated vapours (eg, spraying directly into the mouth) are probably more dangerous than those involving the inhalation of vapor that has been diluted by air. Little is known about the factors affecting long-term risks (if any), but it seems likely that the risk is greatest the larger the amount inhaled, the higher the concentration and the longer the duration of the practice.

A variety of terms have been used to refer to the act of inhaling these products, and, to date, no universally accepted terminology has emerged. The term 'glue sniffing' does not do justice to the range of products that have been abused (quite apart from the fact that they are usually inhaled through the mouth rather than sniffed). The terms 'solvent abuse' and 'solvent misuse' can be criticized on the grounds that some of the products that are inhaled for their intoxicating effects are not solvents (eg. butane) and do not contain chemicals that are used as solvents. American studies have generally employed the term 'inhalants' to refer to this general category of substances. Although there are some advantages to the use of this term, it does not preserve the distinction between products that are made for the purpose of inhaling (eg, certain catarrhal remedies) and those where inhalation represents a deviation from the intended use. The term 'volatile substances' is more accurate, but cumbersome. The term 'solvent abuse' has the advantages and disadvantages of being in colloquial use. In spite of its limitations, it is the term that we shall use for the purposes of this monograph.

1.3 Neurological and Neuropsychological Consequences of Solvent Abuse

1.3.1 Introduction

Concern has frequently been expressed about the potential dangers of solvent abuse. Reports of youngsters dying shortly after sniffing solvents have been widely publicized and worries about the possibility that those who do not die will suffer physical harm have often been voiced.

The risk of sudden death has been well documented both in the USA (Bass, 1970) and the UK (Watson, 1979; Anderson et al, 1985). Approximately half of the recognised fatalities appear to be caused by a direct toxic effect of the solvent, probably on the heart. The other half are attributable to more indirect causes such as aspiration of vomit, plastic bag suffocation, and accidents sustained while intoxicated (Anderson et al, 1985).

In the UK the number of fatalities attributed to solvent abuse rose sharply between 1975 and 1985 (Anderson et al, 1985) such that the practice is now a significant factor in teenage mortality. Nevertheless, in absolute terms, fatalities are still quite rare. Until 1984, for example, the total number of such deaths throughout the UK was less than a hundred per year. If this figure is contrasted with the proportion of young people who have tried abusing solvents, a figure of 4 to 5% in two of the more satisfactory British studies (NOP, 1982; Plant, Peck and Samuel, 1985), it is clear that the vast majority of those who sniff do not die as a result of the practice.

Less is known about the risks of long-term physical harm resulting from solvent abuse. Damage to the liver, kidneys and blood has been reported in several studies, although as Watson (1986) has pointed out, the total number of people reported world-wide as showing persistent toxic effects on the liver and kidneys is rather low. The possibility of long-term damage to the brain has caused particular concern and has been the focus of interest in many reports concerning solvent abuse. The present investigation was conducted primarily in order to examine this issue. The available evidence relevant to the suggestion that solvent abuse may result in persistent neurological and/or neuropsychological impairments is considered below. The evidence has to be considered carefully and in some detail. In the past, those seeking to deter various adolescent 'problem behaviors' have been quick to seize on evidence linking such behaviours with neurological and other disorders. Not infrequently the link has not stood up to rigorous examination, and this has sometimes resulted in the rationale of deterrence being called into question instead of just the particular claims put forward.

1.3.2 Studies of Occupational Exposure to Solvents

Before considering the literature on solvent *abuse*, it is convenient to mention briefly the evidence from studies of people exposed to solvents in the course of their work. A number of investigations, particularly from Sweden and Finland, would appear to provide evidence that occupational exposure to industrial solvents can result in neurological and neuropsychiatric impairment (eg, Axelson, 1976; Mikkelson, 1980; Olsen and Sabroe, 1980), although usually the assessments have been conducted in connection with compensation proceedings. More recent studies, and re-examination of earlier investigations, have tended to weaken rather than strengthen the evidence for a causal link (Baker and Fine, 1986; Lindstrom, Riihimaki and Hanninen, 1984; Waldron, 1986; Cherry, Hutchins, Pace and Waldron, 1985). However, as Ron (1986) points out, the relevance of this evidence to the issue of whether solvent *abuse* causes neurological or neuropsychological impairment is limited by a number of considerations. First, the pattern of exposure is different in the two situations. Occupational exposure usually involves low concentrations over extended periods of time, whereas solvent abuse typically involves occasional, brief exposures to very high concentrations. Second, the types of solvents that have been investigated in studies of occupational exposure are often rather different from those present in abused products. For example, styrene and methylene chloride, which have been studied extensively both in the workplace and the laboratory, are rarely present in abused products. Third, the age at which occupational exposure takes place is different from the age when recreational exposure occurs and it is possible that the long-term consequences are partly dependent upon the maturity of the nervous system. For all of these reasons the evidence from studies of occupational exposure to solvents must be regarded as somewhat tangential to the issue of whether or not solvent abuse causes persistent neurological and neuropsychological sequelae.

1.3.3 Solvent Abuse: Neurological Sequelae

The evidence indicating that solvent abuse may result in neurological impairment has come from reports of single cases or of small groups of cases. In virtually all cases it has been concerned with people whose sniffing history extends over many years.

Three main types of neurological signs have been described. Peripheral neuropathies have been well documented (Prockop, 1979; Hall, Ramsey, Schwartz and Dooken, 1986). n-hexane has been implicated in many of these cases (eg, Korobkin, Ashbury, Sumner and Neilson, 1975; Towfighi, Gonatas, Pleasure, Cooper and McCree, 1976,) but other compounds such as methyl n-butyl ketone (MBK) and methyl ethyl ketone (MEK) would appear to have comparable adverse effects (Altenkirch, Mager, Stoltenburg and Helmbrecht, 1977). The role of toluene and other substances currently found in abused products as possible causes of peripheral neuropathies is uncertain, but Fornazzari, Wilkinson, Kapur and Carlen (1983) have reported two mild cases in a group of 24 chronic toluene sniffers.

With n-hexane and MEK, the clinical signs typically develop two or three months after abuse and show a fairly rapid progression involving a symmetrical and primarily distal motor neuropathy leading to paralysis and muscle atrophy in the legs and sometimes in the arms as well. Head and trunk muscles are not usually affected. Sensory disturbance is manifest as a diminution in perception of pain, touch and vibration with loss of joint position sense (Korobkin et al, 1975; Towfighi et al, 1976). Cranial nerves are usually not impaired. Following discontinuation of sniffing (or removal of the substance implicated) a lag of a few weeks occurs before improvement is observed, possibly because solvents are eliminated only slowly from fatty organs such as the central nervous system. The extent of improvement varies from case to case, but impairment persisting for at least eight or nine months has been noted (Altenkirch et al, 1977). Follow-up over longer periods of time does not appear to have been reported.

Cerebellar signs such as ataxia, dysarthria and tremor were first described by Grabski (1961) in a young man who had abused various substances, but primarily toluene, over a two year period. When followed up some years later, the cerebellar signs were still present but toluene was still being abused and the clinical picture was further complicated by carbon tetrachloride abuse (Knox and Nelson, 1966). Subsequent studies have tended to focus on the issue of whether toluene alone can cause a cerebellar syndrome. Several studies have produced evidence that it can (eg, Boor and Hurtig, 1977; Malm and Lying-Tunell, 1980; Fornazzari et al, 1983).Unfortunately, less attention has been paid to the question of whether cerebellar signs *persist* after discontinuation of sniffing. King, Day, Oliver, Lush and Watson (1981) described one case in whom signs persisted for a year after reported cessation of sniffing, but in other investigations recovery has either been observed over shorter periods of time (eg, Malm and Lying-Tunell, 1980) or, more frequently, has not been studied.

Neuroradiological abnormalities have been found in some solvent abusers but not in other, equally chronic, cases. Fornazzari et al (1983) found a widening of the cerebellar and cerebral sulci and an increase in the size of the ventricular system when 14 chronic abusers were compared with age and sex-matched controls investigated for unrelated neurological complaints. The cerebellar abnormalities were significantly correlated with the presence of clinical neurological signs. Follow-up investigations of this sample could not be conducted, but as Ron (1986) points out, the possibility that neuroradiological abnormalities might shrink with the passage of time during abstinence merits investigation. Schikler, Seitz, Rice and Strader (1982) conducted computed tomography scans on 11 solvent abusers who had all been inhaling products containing toluene for at least ten years. Cerebral atrophy was diagnosed in four of them (on the basis of judgments concerning the enlargement of the ventricular system, basal cistern and convexity sulci) and two of these also appeared to show evidence of cerebellar atrophy. However, neuropathological investigations of cases of this type have not yet been reported and the significance of these neuroradiological signs is therefore difficult to decipher.

Other neurological conditions such as cerebral infarction (Parker, Tarlow and Anderson, 1984) and blindness (Ehyai and Freemon, 1983) have also been reported among chronic solvent abusers, but only in individual cases. The association might therefore be coincidental.

1.3.4 Solvent Abuse: Neuropsychological Sequelae

Instead of using neurological procedures to detect damage to the nervous system following solvent abuse, an alternative strategy has been to use neuropsychological tests.

1.3.4.1 Rationale

The rationale for using psychological tests to detect CNS impairment has been considered in detail elsewhere (Chadwick and Rutter, 1983; Wert and Raulin, 1986 a and b) and will be only briefly considered here.

Contemporary approaches to neuropsychological assessment have evolved over the past 40 years or so, and over this period there have been significant changes in the range and type of measures included in such assessments. Initially, greatest emphasis was placed on the use of single tests to diagnose brain damage. For example, on the Bender Visual-Motor Gestalt Test certain types of rotational error in copying the designs were said to be indicative of organic brain pathology. However, as noted in several reviews published in the early 1960s (eg, Herbert, 1964), the results of these early efforts were generally disappointing. Although many of the tests showed statistically significant differences between groups with and without independently diagnosed brain damage, the considerable overlap in test scores often meant that the misclassification rates were unacceptably high when the tests were applied to individual cases. As investigators became increasingly aware of the variability of the psychological sequelae of organic brain damage, these single test measures fell into disfavor and efforts were redirected toward the development of batteries of tests aimed to identify the *several* patterns of psychological impairment that may stem from brain damage. Halstead (1947) and Reitan (1955) in the US were the pioneers of this approach and many of the batteries in use today have their origins in the Halstead-Reitan Neuropsychological Test Battery.

A large body of evidence has accumulated attesting to the sensitivity of test batteries such as these to the presence of structural damage to the brain. Neuropsychological tests have been shown to be capable of detecting impairment attributable to brain damage even in groups of children with no identifiable abnormalities on a standard neurological examination (Rutter and Chadwick, 1980), and with adults such tests have been used to detect the early stages of various neuropathological processes, such as cerebral neoplasms, dementia or chronic alcohol damage. It has been claimed that the reliability and validity of some test batteries is comparable to that achieved by CT scanning (eg, Filskov and Golstein, 1974; Tsushima and Wedding, 1979; Golden, Moses, Fishburne, Engum, Lewis, Wisniewski, Conley, Berg and Graber, 1981), and although the evidence for these claims is debatable (Chadwick and Rutter, 1983), it certainly is the case that psychological testing is now accepted and used extensively in research to assess the effects of brain injury and disease as well as to examine the effects of central nervous system exposures such as X-irradiation of the brain, elevated lead levels and psychoactive drug use. Their sensitivity, reliability and lack of associated medical risks make them particularly useful in monitoring the effects of these exposures over time.

As well as being one of their main strengths, the sensitivity of psychological tests is also one of their main drawbacks, for in addition to being sensitive to the effects of brain injury, they are affected by other factors, such as age, educational level, socio-economic status and level of motivation. This lack of specificity means that psychological test measures are more liable than neurological tests to yield false-positive findings unless steps are taken to control for the effects of these other factors. Unfortunately, this point has often been neglected in studies investigating the neuropsychological sequelae of solvent abuse.

1.3.4.2 Findings

One of the earliest studies to use neuropsychological tests to examine the effects of solvent abuse was that carried out in Denver by Dodds and Santostefano (1964). A group of 12 boys who had been apprehended by the police for sniffing glue was compared with a control group on a battery of tests of sustained attention, visual memory, visual perception and visuo-motor skills. The two groups differed markedly in terms of ethnic background and were given different tests of general intellectual abilities, but both groups were said to be of average intelligence. No test data are presented, but it was reported that no significant differences between groups were found on any of the test measures. However, the battery of tests that was used had apparently been designed for a purpose other than neuropsychological investigation, and in the absence of validation data, their sensitivity to any damage that may have been present is open to question.

More recent North American investigations have tended to use the Halstead-Reitan neuropsychological test battery and have generally reported significant impairment when groups of chronic solvent abusers have been compared with controls. In a preliminary report of a study to examine the neuropsychological effects of amphetamine abuse as well as solvent abuse, Trites, Suh, Offord, Nieman and Preston (1976) compared a group of 27 solvent abusers with 15 same-sex sibling controls on an extensive battery of tests. Typically, the cases had abused solvents more than twice a day over a period of approximately two years. An attempt was made to exclude those who acknowledged solvent abuse during the two months prior to assessment, although it is unclear from the published report whether blood and urine tests were carried out on the solvent abusers. Both groups were below average on most tests. The solvent abusers had a mean Full Scale IQ four points lower than that of the controls, the deficit in Verbal IQ being greater than in Performance IQ. The results of significance tests are not presented, but relative to the controls the solvent abusers were most noticeably impaired on tests of memory function and timed perceptuo-motor tasks such as the Tactual Performance Test and the Trail-Making test.

Berry, Heaton and Kirby (1977) and Berry (1976) examined a sample of 37 cases aged between 15 and 29 years who had been sniffing solvents frequently over a period of 1.5 to 17 years prior to assessment. Cases were excluded from the sample where there was evidence from self-report, clinical assessment or toxicological examination of urine specimens of sniffing during the preceding 72 hours. The sample was compared with a small control group consisting of siblings or friends of the cases who had never sniffed solvents, but who were closely comparable to them in terms of age, sex, education, ethnic background, recent criminal record and history of drug abuse. The Wechsler Adult Intelligence Scale and the Halstead-Reitan test battery were administered without knowledge of the subjects' status as a case or control. The solvent abusers performed less well on each of the tests and the differences between groups were statistically significant on a number of measures in spite of the small size of the control group. The Full Scale IQ of the solvent abusers was 7.5 points below that of the controls, the deficit in Verbal IQ (8.5 points) being slightly more marked than that in Performance IQ (5.5 points). On the Halstead-Reitan battery, impairment was most marked on tests of memory for prose, tactual performance, maze tracing and grip strength.

These two studies provide two of the more satisfactory sources of evidence to date that solvent abuse may cause neuropsychological impairment. Most of the major methodological pitfalls seem to have been avoided, but nevertheless it should be noted that the control groups in both studies were small, and in the Berry et al investigation, the possibility that unintended bias may have operated in the process of selecting suitable volunteer controls to match with the cases cannot be completely ruled out.

A similar pattern of findings was obtained by Korman, Matthews and Lovitt (1981) in Dallas. Samples of 68 solvent abusers and 41 abusers of other substances were recruited from the clientele of a drug treatment unit and their drug-using friends and siblings. Statistically significant differences between the two groups were found on most of the subtests of the Wechsler scales, on the Reading, Spelling and Arithmetic subtests of the Wide Range Achievement Test, as well as on a few of the 50 or so measures from the Halstead-Reitan battery that were used. As in the Berry et al (1977) study, the difference in Verbal IQ was more pronounced than that observed on the Performance scale. Unfortunately, the study is seriously limited in its usefulness because of major omissions from the report. Virtually no information is given about the frequency and extent of solvent abuse in the cases, nor about how recently they had sniffed. In addition, the comparability of the two groups on other factors that might affect psychological test performance was not considered.

In a study which focused primarily on the neurological status of solvent abusers, Fornazzari et al (1983) examined a group of 24 young men who had abused substances containing toluene for an average duration of six years. Fifteen cases (65%) were categorised as 'neurologically impaired' (on the basis of four or more abnormal neurological signs). This subgroup had abused solvents for longer than the neurologically unimpaired subgroup (approximately 7 years versus 4.5 years on average). The neurologically impaired subgroup were impaired on Verbal IQ, Performance IQ, the Wechsler Memory Scale, a summary measure of performance on the Halstead-Reitan test battery and the Heath Rail Walking Test (a standardized procedure for quantifying ataxic gait). By contrast, the scores of the neurologically unimpaired solvent abusers were normal on all measures except Verbal IQ.

Other studies of the neuropsychological consequences of solvent abuse have been based on samples that are too small to permit reliable conclusions to be drawn.

Tsushima and Towne (1977) found a 20 point difference in IQ between 20 young people who had been sniffing paint for 1 to 13 years and an equal number of controls selected from the same peer and neighbourhood groups. Again, however, precise details of the method of selecting controls were not given. They also found a relationship between the duration of paint sniffing and the magnitude of deficit on a selection of tests from the Halstead-Reitan battery. Four cases who had been involved in sniffing for more than ten years showed poorer performance on the tests than cases with a shorter history of solvent abuse. This finding is consistent with the possibility of a causal effect of solvent abuse on neuropsychological functioning. However, quite apart from the small size of the subsamples, it is possible, as the authors acknowledge, that those with a longer history of drug abuse may have been less educationally able in the first place.

Bigler (1979) compared a group of ten solvent abusers with equal sized groups of psychotic, non-psychotic and brain damaged patients at a State Hospital in Austin, Texas. All of the patients were reported to be very disturbed. The solvent abusers performed significantly less well than the non-psychotic patients on the Wechsler scales and parts of the Halstead Reitan battery, and their performance on these tests was in general not significantly different from that of the psychotic and brain damaged patients. The solvent abusers appeared to be most impaired on tests of Verbal IQ, concept attainment and tactual performance, but the results of this study do not inspire great confidence, partly because of the small sample sizes, but more particularly because most of the solvent abusers were taking neuroleptic drugs at the time of the assessment.

Studies from the UK have generally used more circumscribed batteries of tests and have produced more equivocal findings. Mahmood (1983), in Glasgow, obtained a mixed and rather puzzling pattern of results when 28 solvent abusers attending a clinic were compared with 20 secondary school children who were said to be comparable in terms of age and socio-economic background. The solvent abusers performed significantly worse than the controls on tests of vocabulary and reading ability, but obtained significantly higher scores than the controls on tests of arithmetic and verbal learning.

Zur and Yule (1990, a) compared a sample of 12 solvent abusers identified from a number of different sources with an equal number of delinquent controls recruited from a Regional Assessment Centre. The two groups consisted only of boys and were comparable in terms of years spent in full-time education, history of delinquency and parental alcoholism, employment status and prison record. A wide variety of different solvents had been abused by the cases, but all of them had sniffed glue and the majority had also abused typewriter correction fluids. Their history of solvent abuse ranged from 1.5 to 5 years. All of them had sniffed at least four or five times a week. The two groups were compared on the Wechsler Scales and a battery of computerised tests including measures of visual discrimination, perception of spatial orientation, verbal and visual recognition memory and serial choice reaction time. No significant differences between the solvent abusers and their controls were found on the Wechsler subtests. On the computerized battery of tests, the solvent abusers made significantly more errors on the choice reaction time and visual discrimination tasks after controlling for differences in age between the two groups. However, testing was carried out after a period of abstinence of only 24 hours, and toxicological examination of blood and urine samples carried out on five of the cases showed that all five were positive for toluene. It therefore remains possible that the observed deficits reflect on acute, rather than a long-term, effect of solvent abuse.

In most of the studies of solvent abuse described above, the cases and controls were selected from different sources. A small unpublished study conducted by Raczka (1983) is different in this respect in as much as both groups were sampled from the same source: a Community Home for young offenders. One major advantage of selecting both samples from the same source is that this decreases the likelihood of adventitious background differences between groups on variables hat might affect psychological test performance. All of the boys who were attending a school within the grounds of the Home were assessed: 14 solvent abusers and 15 non-sniffing controls. The two groups were comparable in terms of age, time since first delinquent offense, period of detention and parental employment status. All of the cases reported regular abuse of a toluene-containing glue, but other volatile substances had also been abused occasionally. Their history of abuse ranged from one to five years with an estimated average weekly consumption of two litres. None of them reported having abused solvents during the three days prior to assessment (although no toxicological examination was done to verify these reports). The two groups were given an abbreviated version of the Wechsler Scales and a battery of neuropsychological tests to measure finger tapping speed, impulsivity, susceptibility to distraction and memory. In addition, the New Adult Reading Test was administered to provide an estimate of 'premorbid' functioning. The tests were administered before information about solvent abuse was collected in order to maintain blindness to the subjects status as a case or control. No significant differences between groups were found at the 1% level of chance on any of the test measures. Similarly, the correlations between test performance and total lifetime consumption of solvent (estimated from the duration of sniffing and the average amount sniffed) were inconsistent and not statistically significant.

Allison and Jerrom (1984) also identified their cases and controls from the same source. They interviewed a population of 65 adolescent boys at three residential schools for offenders in the West of Scotland. Eighty percent of them had sniffed glue or other volatile substances and the ten cases with the most serious history of sniffing were compared with ten non-abusing controls selected from the same school as the cases. The two groups were said to be comparable in terms of age, educational level and reading age (although no educational test results were presented). They were compared on a short battery of tests consisting of the vocabulary and block design subtests of the Wechsler Scales, the Wechsler Memory Scale and a test of paced serial addition. The solvent abusers showed significant impairment on all tests except vocabulary and two of the seven subtests of the Memory Scale. Although this pattern of test results is suggestive of neuropsychological impairment, as the authors point out, no toxicological examination was performed to confirm the boys' reports that none of them had sniffed during the ten days prior to assessment.

1.3.4.3 Conclusion

It is not possible to reach any firm conclusions about the neuropsychological consequences of solvent abuse on the basis of the studies considered above. Their findings have been rather inconsistent, with some investigators reporting no deficits in psychological test performance (eg, Dodds and Santostefano, 1964; Raczka, 1983), and others finding marked impairment at least on some measures (eg, Tsushima and Towne, 1979; Mahmood, 1983; Bigler, 1979). However, comparison between the findings of the different studies is made difficult because many of them suffer from quite serious limitations in design, execution or reporting. A number of different methodological problems may be identified. First, almost all of the investigations have used samples that are far too small for confidence to be placed in their findings. Second, in many studies far too little attention has been paid to the importance of ensuring comparability between cases and controls on factors other than solvent abuse. Third, several investigations have failed to take adequate steps to ensure that the cases were not under the acute influence of solvents at the time of psychological testing. Fourth, in only two of the studies has testing been carried out 'blind' to the subject's status as a case or control. (This might not matter particularly if all of the tests used were computerised, as there would then be little opportunity for any possible examiner bias to operate, but all of the studies have used some non-computerized tests.) Fifth, these methodological problems have sometimes been compounded by deficiencies in reporting: in several studies important details of the methods used or the results have been omitted. For example, some reports have failed to provide an indication of how often or for how long the cases had abused solvents. Finally, in studies where where significant differences between cases and controls have been found, insufficient attention has been paid to the possibility that impairment was due to factors other than solvent abuse.

1.4 Additional Issues to be Addressed in the Study

Although the main concern of the present investigation is with the *effects* of solvent abuse, the design of the study made it possible to investigate two other major issues concerning solvent abuse at the same time. These are (a) the prevalence and pattern of solvent abuse among secondary school children, and (b) the socio-demographic characteristics of solvent abusers and the correlates of the practice. Evidence bearing on these two issues is briefly reviewed below.

1.4.1 The Prevalence and Pattern of Solvent Abuse Among Secondary School Children

Although a number of studies to examine the prevalence of solvent abuse have been conducted in North America, information on the prevalence among young people in Britain is currently limited. Prior to the end of the last decade, only a few isolated surveys had been conducted to examine the use of illicit drugs by school children and none of these had enquired specifically about solvents (Stimson, 1981). Since then, a limited amount of information has become available. In 1979, Plant and his colleagues (1985) examined the extent of alcohol and drug use by means of a self-completed questionnaire that was administered to over 1000 fifth year (15 to 16 year old) pupils attending five schools in Edinburgh and the surrounding Lothian region. The schools were selected so as to be representative of school leavers in the region. Just under one in twenty (4.6%) indicated that they had tried glues, solvents or dry-cleaning agents at some time in the past. Of the illicit drugs, only cannabis (7.2%) and tranquilizers (5.2%) had been used by a higher proportion of the sample.

Consistent with the findings of this study are the results of a 1982 survey conducted by NOP Market Research Ltd of a representative sample of over 1000 British 15 to 21 year olds. Among the 15 and 16 year olds who were questioned, 4.3% acknowledged that they had sniffed glue. The proportion indicating that they had done so 'often' was only 0.5%. Several unpublished local surveys of schools in different parts of the UK have also been conducted (Institute for the Study of Drug Dependence, 1986) and these have tended to yield higher rates of reported solvent abuse than the two studies discussed above. For example, in 1983, 8.1% of 11 to 18 year olds at 9 schools in East Sussex indicated that they had abused solvents during the preceding year (Faber, 1985), and in a Berkshire survey 8.5% of school children said they had tried sniffing (Lynch, 1984). While there is good evidence indicating that the rate of solvent abuse varies from place to place and from time to time, the higher rates obtained in these ad hoc local surveys cannot be accepted without reservation because of the possibility that schools with high levels of drug and solvent abuse were preferentially approached for permission to conduct the survey.

Nevertheless, recent published studies have also tended to yield higher prevalence rates. For example, Swadi (1988) administered a questionnaire to a sample of 3333 11 to 16 year old pupils attending six Inner London comprehensive schools and found that 11% acknowledged solvent abuse. Diamond, Pritchard, Choudry, Fielding, Cox and Bushnell (1988) found the prevalence of solvent abuse among 4th and 5th year pupils (aged 14 to 16) at six schools in Southampton and Bournemouth was 12.5% in 1985 and 8.8% when the survey was repeated in 1986. Again however, in both of these studies, few details of the method of selecting schools were presented. This problem does not apply to the study conducted by Cooke, Evans and Farrow (1988) who administered a questionnaire to a one in six sample of pupils on the registers of 28 of the 29 maintained secondary schools in one county of South Wales in 1985. Completed questionnaires were obtained from 4474 pupils, 90.9% of the target population, making this one of the largest and most comprehensive studies undertaken so far. 6.8% admitted to having abused solvents, although as in other population-based surveys, approximately half of these cases had sniffed only once.

A subsidiary aim of the present study was to supplement these findings by examining the prevalence of solvent abuse in an unselected sample of urban school children.

1.4.2 Socio-demographic and Clinical Characteristics of Solvent Abusers

Early case reports and case series from the United States consistently reported that males were over represented among solvent abusers (Lawton and Malmquist, 1961; Sterling, 1964; Press and Done, 1967). They also indicated an excess of children from large families (Barker and Adams, 1963), often living in impoverished circumstances (Sokol and Robinson, 1963). Broken homes and parental alcoholism were common (Brozovsky and Winkler, 1965; Massengale, Glaser, LeLievre, Dodds and Klock, 1963) and the children themselves were claimed to show poor educational attainments (Ackerly and Gibson, 1964; Press and Done, 1967).

However, in all of these early studies the samples consisted of collections of youngsters who had been apprehended by the police or referred for psychiatric evaluation or treatment for solvent abuse. Delinquents and other adolescents with conduct disorders are likely to be overrepresented among these groups. The findings may therefore merely reflect the recognized relationships between delinquency and male sex, large family size, low socio-economic status, broken homes and poor educational attainment found in many studies of juvenile delinquents (Rutter and Giller, 1983), rather than an association specific to solvent abuse. More representative samples of solvent abusers are needed if generalizations of this type are to be valid.

The present study provided the opportunity to investigate the links between solvent abuse and these socio-demographic and clinical factors in a representative sample of adolescents attending secondary schools. This was the second subsidiary aim of the study.

1.5   Rationale of the Design of the Present Investigation

All of the evidence reviewed earlier concerning the effects of solvent abuse has come from studies of clinic referrals who have abused solvents heavily and usually over prolonged periods of time. The findings of such studies cannot necessarily be generalized to samples whose pattern and history of solvent abuse is different. In the present investigation, an attempt was made to investigate the effects of the practice at frequencies prevalent among secondary school children. A population-based survey was used to provide a sampling frame for the selection of 'exposed' cases and 'unexposed' controls, and the neuropsychological status of these two groups was then compared.

A number of methodological problems were noted above in reviewing previous studies of the neuropsychological consequences of solvent abuse. The ways in which these problems were addressed in the present study are discussed below.

1.5.1 Sample Size

Most previous studies have been carried out on samples that are too small to inspire confidence in the findings: most have relied on samples of fewer than 20 cases. In the present investigation, more than 100 matched case-control pairs were compared. This provided an 80% chance of detecting a difference between groups of 0.40 standard deviations and a 90% chance of detecting a difference of 0.46 standard deviations, assuming that an effect exists.

1.5.2 Comparability of Cases and Controls on Factors Other than Solvent Abuse

In most previous studies of the neuropsychological sequelae of solvent abuse, the cases and controls have been selected from different sources. The cases have typically been selected from those referred for psychological assessment and treatment, whereas the controls have been selected from a variety of other sources. The selection of the two groups from different populations, increases the likelihood of adventitious background differences between groups on variables that might affect psychological test performance.

In the present investigation, the controls were selected from the same broadly defined population of secondary school attenders as the cases and two groups were also individually matched for school, school year and sex. Since performance on neuropsychological tests may be affected by factors such as socio-economic status or ethnic origin (Prigitano and Parsons, 1976; Finlayson, Johnson and Reitan, 1977), and since there is evidence indicating that solvent abusers differ from non-abusers on these variables it was necessary to devise a way of controlling for these factors. Further matching on parental socioeconomic status and ethnic background was not attempted in the present study because cases and controls were matched before they were interviewed and it was considered impractical, if not objectionable, to try and obtain this information on the screening questionnaire. Instead, statistical techniques were used to control for the effects of any observed background differences between groups. Detailed information was collected on a range of social factors in order to ensure that the effects of background differences between groups on psychological test performance could be controlled statistically.

1.5.3 Acute Intoxication

One of the worries about many previous investigations of the effects of solvent abuse has been that, because objective measures to detect current intoxication have rarely been included, it has not been possible to reject the hypothesis that the cases were intoxicated, or at least still subject to the acute effects of solvents, at the time the psychological tests were administered. In order to ensure that the present study was concerned with the *long-term* effects of solvent abuse rather than the immediate effects of intoxication, it was necessary to be able to detect and, if necessary, exclude those children who were under the acute influence of solvents (or alcohol) at the time of testing. This was done by analyzing breath samples from each child immediately after completion of the psychological tests by means of a technique that utilized mass spectrometry to detect and identify trace levels of volatile compounds in exhaled air.

1.5.4 Blindness

Although 'blindness' to the child's status as a case or control is not as crucial an issue as it is when assessment depends on subjective ratings or judgments, there are advantages to administering the psychological tests without knowledge of group membership. The main advantage is that it provides an extra degree of reassurance that the findings are unlikely to be influenced by any possible experimenter bias. In the present study, the complete battery of psychological tests was therefore administered in ignorance of the reason for the child's selection for detailed assessment and without knowledge of his or her questionnaire, interview and toxicological exam findings.

1.5.5 The Choice of Measures to Assess Outcome

In view of the paucity and inconsistency in the evidence to date on the *types* of psychological sequelae likely to be present among solvent abusers, an extensive battery of tests examining a range of different psychological functions was used in the present study. Some tests were selected on the basis of their demonstrated sensitivity to the effects of prolonged solvent abuse or occupational exposure to solvents. Others were selected on the basis of their sensitivity to chronic alcohol abuse in adults. Studies documenting the neuropsychological sequelae of various types of acquired brain injury in childhood (due to meningitis or head injury, for example) also contributed to the rationale for test selection.

1.5.6 Test Performance Antecedent to Solvent Abuse

If solvent abuse *causes* psychological impairment, it follows that not only should the impairment be present in those with a history of solvent abuse, but also that the impairment should not have been present at the same level prior to the beginning of that history. In order to provide a measure of ability *antecedent* to solvent abuse in the present study, the results of all standardised educational tests that had been administered at or before the time of transfer from primary to secondary school were obtained from the schools. The child's current test performance could therefore be compared with his or her performance prior to solvent abuse, thus making it possible to examine whether the performance of the cases had deteriorated since they started sniffing. These data also made it possible to take account statistically of any differences between groups in ability antecedent to solvent abuse.

2 Method

2.1 Summary

A sample of children who had abused solvents was identified by means of a self-completed screening questionnaire that was administered to the third, fourth and fifth year pupils (ages 13 to 16 years) at sixteen secondary schools.

At each school, a sample of those who acknowledged that they had inhaled solvents to the point of intoxication at any time in the past were selected for individual assessment. For each case, a control who denied sniffing on the questionnaire was also selected. The controls were selected from the same schools as the cases and were individually matched for school year and sex.

The individual assessments consisted of a short interview, a breath test and an extensive battery of psychological tests.

The purpose of the interview was to validate the child's questionnaire responses, to obtain detailed information on the frequency and pattern of solvent abuse, and to collect information on background socio-demographic and other factors that might be expected to affect psychological test performance.

The aim of the breath test was to identify children who might have been under the influence of solvents (or alcohol) at the time of psychological testing.

The battery of neuropsychological tests was designed to assess a range of functions implicated in previous studies of (a) chronic solvent abuse or occupational exposure to solvents, or (b) other CNS exposures, such as alcohol abuse in adults or severe head injury or meningitis in children and adolescents. It included measures of general intellectual and reading ability as well as tests to assess more specific functions such as psychomotor speed, attention, memory, manual and digital dexterity, and vibration perception.

In order to permit longitudinal comparisons with test results prior to solvent abuse, the schools were asked to provide details of the results of any standardized educational tests that had been taken by the cases and controls at or before the time of transfer from primary to secondary school.

During the following school year, follow-up assessments were conducted in order to provide longitudinal data on the practice of solvent abuse, to examine the stability of the psychological test findings from the initial assessment and to supplement the range of measures used at the initial assessment. Children who had been individually assessed and who were still at school were retraced and reexamined on questionnaires and a similar battery of psychological tests.

2.2 The Target Population

Permission to conduct the study in local authority secondary schools was requested and obtained from the Directors of Education of four local education authorities: one division of the Inner London Education Authority (area A) and three outer London boroughs (areas B, C and D). In areas A and B, the schools were selected by the research team on the basis of their geographical location: an attempt was made to sample schools from as many different parts of these areas as possible.

In areas C and D, they were selected by the borough Education Departments. Following an introductory letter, a senior member of the research team visited the Headteacher (or Deputy Head) in order to explain the study, seek permission to conduct it and make arrangements to do so. Twenty four schools were approached and 20 of them agreed to participate: five from area A, eight from area B, three from area C and four from area D. Four schools in area A declined to participate.

Pilot studies were conducted at the four schools in area D during the school year 1983-4. These studies were used to test and develop the survey instruments and procedures and to collect preliminary data on solvent abuse in the area of investigation. As a result of these studies, it was decided to restrict the target population to third year (aged 13 to 14 years), fourth year (aged 14 to 15 years) and fifth year (aged 15 to 16 years) pupils.

The study proper was conducted at the 16 schools in areas A, B and C. In one school the study was conducted during the school year 1983-4, but in the other 15 schools it was carried out during the autumn, spring and summer terms of the school year 1984-5. Seven of the schools were coeducational and nine were single-sex schools (five for girls only, four for boys only). Table 3 provides summary details of the sex and year groups surveyed at each of the schools. The target population consisted of 40 school year groups. Fourth year pupils (aged 14 to 15 years) were surveyed at all 16 schools. Third year pupils (aged 13 to 14 years) were surveyed at 12 of the schools but not at the other four. (Three of them did not admit children younger than 14 at the time the study was conducted and at the fourth it was not possible to include the 3rd year pupils because of scheduling difficulties.) Fifth year pupils (aged 15 to 16 years) were also surveyed at 12 of the 16 schools. They were omitted at the other four schools where the questionnaire survey was conducted during the summer term. Their omission was deliberate. Many fifth year pupils elect to leave school at Easter and those who stay on to take public examinations during the summer term are therefore likely to be unrepresentative of fifth year pupils in general.

2.3 Parental Permission and Absentees

Shortly before the questionnaire was due to be administered at each school, letters to the parents of each child were delivered to the school office in sealed envelopes. The letter explained in general terms the aims of the study and what would be involved. The parents were requested to complete a tear-off slip and return it to the school office if they did *not* wish their child to take part. The schools made their own arrangements for the pupils to address the envelopes to their parents. Arrangements for delivering the letter differed from school to school according to the policy of the Headteacher. At ten of the schools the children were told to take the sealed letter home and deliver it by hand to their parents. At five schools the addressed letters were collected by a member of the research team, stamped and then mailed to the parents. At one school (No. 12), at the request of the Headteacher, the letter was redrafted as an announcement informing the parents that all fourth and fifth year pupils would be taking part in a health study that was being conducted by St George's Hospital.

As shown in Table 3, 7485 pupils were listed on the school registers of the classes that comprised the target population. 825 (11.0%) of them were excluded at the request of their parents or guardians and 1180 (15.8%) were officially recorded as absent on the morning or afternoon the questionnaire was administered. Some of the absentees were children whose parents had refused permission for them to take part in the study, but the degree of the overlap between these two groups is unknown.

2.4 The Screening Questionnaire

2 050

The primary objective of the self-completed screening questionnaire was to identify children who had abused solvents or other volatile substances at any time in the past.

In designing the questionnaire, it was thought that there might be difficulties in obtaining the cooperation of the schools and truthful responses from the pupils if the questions were perceived as being concerned solely with a socially disapproved activity like solvent abuse. In view of this, an attempt was made to dilute the impact of the questions on solvents by embedding them among items concerned with other aspects of general and respiratory health.

The wording and layout of the questionnaire were refined over the course of four pilot studies involving nearly 2000 pupils from schools in borough D. The final version (shown in Appendix A) began with eight items concerned with age, sex and domestic circumstances. These were followed by six questions relating to general and respiratory health. The items dealing with cigarette smoking, solvent sniffing and alcohol consumption came next, and these were followed by a fifteen part question concerned with various behavioural aspects of health. The questionnaire finished with two relatively neutral items focusing attention on physical exercise. Space was provided at the end for comments.

The idea of including questions on the use of drugs such as cannabis, LSD, cocaine and heroin was considered but eventually rejected in order to reduce the length of the questionnaire, to enhance its acceptability to the schools and to facilitate, as far as possible, a 'low profile' in conducting the study.

Because the main purpose of the questionnaire was to select children for further and more detailed assessment, it was necessary to have some means of identifying individual respondents. Two methods were piloted. For the first two pilot studies, everyone was asked to write their names in a space provided at the front of the questionnaire. For the third and fourth pilot studies, they were required to record their school class and date of birth; those selected for the detailed assessments were subsequently identified using the school register. This latter method was found to be workable and preferable. Although a few children could not be traced (presumably because they had recorded an incorrect date of birth), the anonymity almost certainly helped bring to light a number of other children who would have been missed if they had been required to record their names on the questionnaire. This method was therefore used at each of the sixteen schools that participated in the study proper.

At each school, prior to the date of the questionnaire survey, a timetable was prepared by a member of the school staff that would enable the research team to administer the questionnaire to all of the pupils that were to be surveyed. The questionnaire took about 15 to 25 minutes for each child to complete and it was therefore possible to administer it to each group during the course of a single school lesson. At all except one of the schools, it was administered to each class in their normal classrooms, usually by a single member of the research team. By employing this method of screening, four members of the research team were able to complete the screening of the three year groups during the course of the school day. (A different procedure was followed at school No. 14: at the request of the headteacher, the questionnaire was administered in the school assembly hall where each school year was surveyed 'en masse', one at a time).

The survey was introduced to the children by a member of the research team and it was explained that the questionnaire was concerned with various things that might affect the health of young people. The confidentiality of the child's questionnaire responses was explained and the children were encouraged to seek advice from the person administering it if they were unsure about how to answer any of the questions. To emphasise confidentiality, the teachers were openly encouraged to feel free to leave the classroom as soon as the children had settled.

As shown in Table 3, completed questionnaires were obtained from a total of 5014 pupils at the 16 participating schools. The number of completed questionnaires is smaller than the number of children who were officially present in school when the questionnaire was administered and whose parents gave permission for them to take part. This is because (a) a few children may have left the school premises after registering but before doing the questionnaire, (b) some of the children refused to complete the questionnaire, and (c) at a few schools the timetable was such that it was not possible to survey all classes in the target year groups. When this happened, it was not always possible to determine how many children had been missed.

2.5 The Individual Assessments

Positive and negative respondents to the questionnaire items on solvent abuse were scheduled for detailed individual assessment. The individual assessments consisted of three main parts: a short interview, a breath test and an extensive battery of psychological tests.

2.5.1 Selection of Children for Individual Assessment

Those who answered "yes" to the questions "Have you ever sniffed glue, solvents or anything else on purpose?" and "Have you ever sniffed enough to feel 'high' or intoxicated?" on the self-completed questionnaire were eligible for individual assessment as potential cases. Those who answered "no" to the first of these questions were eligible for individual assessment as potential controls. The negative questionnaire respondents were selected from the same schools as the positive questionnaire respondents and were individually matched for school year and sex.

The completed questionnaires were examined by an administrative assistant who did not participate in the individual assessments. Positive questionnaire respondents who indicated frequent solvent abuse on the questionnaire (and their controls) were scheduled for individual assessment before those who indicated that they had abused solvents less often. This was done in order to ensure that as many frequent abusers as possible were tested in the time available at each school (usually not more than a week) and thus to enable the study to test the null hypothesis (of no neuropsychological impairment due to solvent abuse) at the high frequency end of the normal spectrum of abuse.

The individual assessments were conducted at the schools and were arranged to take place as soon as possible after the questionnaire had been administered usually on the next school day). The administrative assistant who examined the questionnaires was also responsible for identifying the selected children by means of the school registers and for finding and escorting them to the assessment rooms. Positive and negative questionnaire respondents were scheduled for individual assessment in quasi-random order, so as not to compromise the examiners' blindness to the child's questionnaire response. The psychological tests and interviews were administered by two other members of the research team working in parallel and in separate rooms. As soon as testing and interviewing had been completed, the child was escorted to a third room where a fourth member of the team conducted the toxicological examination, administered the respiratory tests, measured the child's height and took vibration perception threshold measurements.

Each component of the detailed assessments was carried out without knowledge of (a) the child's questionnaire responses, and (b) the findings from the other components of the detailed assessments. The only exception to this rule was the interview, which was given immediately after the psychological tests and by the same member of the research team. The interviews were therefore conducted after the child's psychological test performance had been observed and recorded.

2.5.2 The Interview
The purpose of the interview was (a) to provide a means of validating the child's questionnaire responses to the items on solvent abuse, (b) to obtain detailed information on the frequency and pattern of solvent abuse, (c) to collect information on background, sociodemographic and other factors that might be expected to affect psychological test performance, and (d) to collect information about the recent use of prescribed medicines (such as asthma inhalers) and other exposures that might affect the toxicological findings.

Although the interview questions were asked in a standard order using a standard form of wording, the interviewers were encouraged to supplement the basic interview schedule in any way they judged likely to set the child at ease and thereby ncrease the chances of obtaining valid and truthful information. Children differ in their willingness to provide information particularly about proscribed behaviors and it was therefore left to the individual interviewer to continue questioning until an adequate account had been obtained.

The interview schedule started with a series of questions to obtain identifying and background information relating to the child's age, family, domestic circumstances and parental employment. These were followed by questions about the child's current and past health as reflected by his or her history of serious illnesses, hospitalisations, accidents, injuries and current use of prescribed medicines (including asthma inhalers). Next were two questions concerned with the proximity of the child's home to sources of air pollution and these were immediately followed by detailed questions on current and past cigarette smoking and history of solvent sniffing. In addition to questions on whether the child had sniffed and whether intoxication had been achieved, this latter section included items concerned with the products that had been sniffed, the frequency, method and most recent occasion of sniffing, the length of time since the child had started to sniff, whether they sniffed alone or in company and where they went to sniff. This was followed by questions on alcohol consumption and drunkenness. The interview finished with questions about the child's school progress, relationships with teachers, school-leaving and career plans.

2.5.3 Toxicological Examination

The purpose of the toxicological assessment was to detect and identify volatile substances present in the child's breath, and thereby to identify those who may have been under the influence of volatile substances (or alcohol) at the time of psychological testing.

Analysis of breath samples was carried out by means of a Personnel and Environmental Trace Gas Analyser (PETRA - VG Instruments, Cheshire), which utilizes mass spectrometry to measure trace levels of volatile substances in exhaled air. It was set to cycle over eight different mass/charge (m/z) ratios, which were selected on the basis of their sensitivity and specificity to volatile compounds likely to be found in abused products. The compounds that could be identified by means of this technique are shown in Table 4.

Subjects were tested one at a time. Each child was seated and asked to take a deep breath and exhale into the breath sampling tube. The output on channel 1 (m/z 46: carbon dioxide) was observed to check that a valid breath sample (of deep alveolar air) had been obtained. If unsatisfactory, a further breath sample was requested.

An initial coarse screen was carried out to determine whether the output of any of the eight channels was elevated. If a response was obtained, a further breath sample was taken and scanned for different fragments in order to identify the compound present. A complete mass spectrum (from m/z 1 to 200) of the breath sample was also recorded.

The maximum output on each of the eight selected channels was recorded on magnetic disk for later analysis. The output was also displayed on an eight - channel chart recorder to provide an immediate visual indication of the findings.

In addition, the presence of alcohol was tested for using an Infra-red Analyser (Camic, Northumberland), but was not detected in the breath of any child.

2.5.4 Neuropsychological Assessment

In view of the contradictory nature of the findings from previous studies of solvent abuse, the battery of neuropsychological tests was designed to assess a range of functions rather than concentrate on a few specific aspects of mental performance. Some of the tests were selected on the basis of evidence that they were sensitive to the effects of chronic solvent abuse or occupational exposure to solvents. Others were selected on the basis of evidence that the functions they assessed were sensitive to the effects of the CNS damage due to exposures, such as chronic alcohol abuse in adults, and severe head injury or meningitis in children and adolescents.

The tests are listed below and are described in detail in Appendix B. They took approximately one and a half hours to complete and were administered without knowledge of the child's questionnaire, interview or toxicological findings. Some of the tests were administered using Apple IIe microcomputers with a special response console: these are indicated by an asterisk.

Wechsler Intelligence Scale for Children - Revised (Wechsler, 1974)
    Similarities
    Vocabulary
    Picture Completion
    Block Design

EH-3 Reading Test (Bate, 1970)

Passage Recall
    Immediate and delayed recall
Speed of information processing (Version E) from the British Ability Scales (Elliot, Murray and Pearson, 1983)
Bexley-Maudsley Automated Psychological Tests (Acker and Acker, 1982)
    * Visual Perceptual Analysis
    * Symbol-Digit Coding Test
Automated Psychological Test System (Elithorn and Levander, unpublished)
    * Reaction Time Tasks
    * Finger Tapping Task
    * Trail-Making Tasks
Manual Dexterity Task (Annett, 1970)
Vibration Perception Threshold Measurement: Thumb and ankle

24

2.5.5 Lung Function Testing

Since inhalation is the route by which solvents are taken in, it seemed important to carry out a simple test of ventilatory capacity which might detect damage to the airways. Ventilatory capacity was measured with a spirometer (Vitalograph) and recorded as forced expiratory volume in one second ($FEV_{1.0}$) and forced vital capacity (FVC). The procedure followed that recommended by the American Thoracic Society (1979). The standing subject was required to breath in as far as possible then blow as hard and as long as possible into the spirometer. A trace of volume against time was obtained from which the FEV and FVC were measured. Following two practice blows, the procedure was carried out three times, and the highest value was recorded. Another measure of ventilatory capacity, the peak expiratory flow rate (PEFR), was measured using a Wright Peak Flow meter.

2.6 Information Obtained from the Schools

2.6.1 Test Performance Prior to Solvent Abuse

In order to obtain information on educational test performance *antecedent* to solvent abuse, the schools were asked to provide details of the results on any standardized educational tests that had been taken by the cases and controls at or before the time of transfer from primary to secondary school. With the cases, the date when the test was taken was compared with the age when the child had started to abuse solvents (as determined at interview) to ensure that the test had indeed been taken prior to solvent abuse. With three children, it was not possible to confirm that this had been the case, and the educational test data for these cases were therefore rejected.

Valid data came from (a) tests of reading ability (Neale Analysis of Reading Ability, Schonell Word Reading Test, Holborn Reading Test, London Reading Test or Burt Word Reading Test) or (b) verbal reasoning tests (National Foundation for Educational Research VR Tests, Cognitive Abilities Test (VQ) and the Moray House VR Test). On most of the tests, the data came in the form of an age standardized quotient with a mean of 100 and a standard deviation of 15, but on the Neale, Schonell and Holborn reading tests, the scores came in the form of a reading age (in years and months). In order to convert these two types of score to the same metric, the reading ages were transformed into equivalent scores on the London Reading Test (Form A) using the empirical data collected to validate the test (London Reading Test, 1980; Table 5), and then converted into standardized quotients.

2.6.2 School Attendance

Although the self-completed questionnaire included an item concerned with how often the adolescent had "stayed away from school or left early" when he or she should have been there, it was considered useful also to try and obtain data on school attendance from the school registers. Attendance data were obtained from all of the schools except one, where the building that housed the registers had been burned down. The number of half-days on which the cases and controls at each of the schools had been officially recorded as (a) late and (b) absent for registration during an arbitrarily selected four week period in November 1984 was recorded. (At all but three of the schools the initial assessments took place later than this four week period.) It had been hoped that it would be possible to distinguish between justified absences (due, for example, to illness or staff industrial action) and unjustified absences, but at some schools this distinction was found difficult to apply and the two were eventually pooled together.

2.7 Definition and Composition of the Case and Control Groups

To be counted as cases, the positive questionnaire respondents had to confirm that they had abused solvents to the point of intoxication at interview. To be counted as controls, the negative questionnaire respondents had to deny solvent sniffing at interview.

Figure 1 shows how the case and control groups were derived from the sample of 5014 children who completed the screening questionnaire. Individual assessments were carried out on 132 of the 208 positive questionnaire respondents and solvent abuse was confirmed at interview in 105 of them. Sixteen children who gave an ambiguous response to the questionnaire items on solvent abuse were also interviewed as potential cases, but only one of them confirmed solvent abuse at interview - a boy who had crossed out his initially positive response and changed it to negative. One hundred and thirteen of the 4610 negative questionnaire respondents were interviewed as potential controls and each of them denied solvent abuse at interview. One hundred and six of these 113 were individually matched with a case. The other seven were omitted from the control group.

The total number of interview-confirmed cases and controls was therefore 106 matched pairs. On toxicological examination, seven of the cases and one of the controls were found to be positive for volatile substances in breath. (This finding will be examined and discussed in detail later.) The seven cases on whom toxicology was positive were retained in the sample of cases pending further analysis of the data. The control who was positive was excluded, as was the case with whom he had been matched. The remaining 105 matched pairs form the two groups which will be compared in examining the effect of solvent abuse on neuropsychological functioning.

Table 5 shows the comparability of the cases and controls on the matching variables. In both groups there were 44 boys and 61 girls. Twenty were from the third year, 61 were from the fourth year and 24 were from the fifth year when the individual assessments were conducted. Ninety five of the case-control pairs were matched for school, but for a variety of practical reasons, the other ten cases and controls, although matched for sex and school year, came from different schools.

2.8 The Follow-up Assessment

Follow-up assessments were conducted during the autumn and spring terms of the school year 1985-6. An attempt was made to re-examine all of the cases and controls who had been third and fourth year pupils (aged 13 to 15 years) at the time of the initial assessments (the school year 1984-5). Those who had been 5th year students (aged 15 to 16 years) at the time of the initial assessments were not included in the follow-up target sample because of the likelihood that those continuing at school into the sixth form might be more academically able than those who left, and hence unrepresentative of the total sample of former fifth year pupils.

Parental permission to conduct the follow-up was requested in the letter sent to the parents prior to the initial assessments and was therefore implicit in their earlier consent to the child's participation in the study.

The follow-up assessments were carried out at the same schools and usually in the same rooms as had been used for the initial assessments. Because the examiners were familiar with the names of the cases and controls from the initial assessments, it was not possible to conduct the follow-up assessments 'blind' to the child's status as a case or control, and so wherever possible, they were seen by the same examiner as before in order to promote rapport.

The follow-up assessments consisted of an individually administered self-completed questionnaire dealing with drug and solvent use and a battery of psychological tests similar to that used in the initial assessments. Both of these were administered by the same examiner. Toxicological examinations were not conducted at follow-up (a) because of the small number of positive identifications at the initial assessment, and (b) because preliminary analysis of the data from these assessments had indicated that whether or not the cases with positive toxicology findings were included had little discernible effect on the neuropsychological test results.

2.8.1 The Self-completed Solvent and Drug Use Questionnaire

An individually administered self-completed questionnaire was used to ascertain the child's use of solvents during the interval between the initial and follow-up assessments. This was preferred to an interview assessment because, as explained above, the follow-up assessments were not conducted 'blind', and it was felt that it would be difficult to avoid bias in the degree of thoroughness with which the children were questioned if the examiner was aware of the child's prior history of solvent abuse. The questionnaire was administered at the end of the assessment after all of the psychological tests had been done. It included questions about the use of cigarettes, alcohol and solvents during the interval between the initial and follow-up assessments, and the use of cannabis, amphetamines, cocaine, heroin and 'any other drugs' at any time in the past.

2.8.2 The Follow-up Neuropsychological Assessment Battery

Several changes were made to the psychological test battery for the follow-up assessment. Some of the tests used at the initial assessment was retained so that initial and follow-up results could be compared, but others were replaced or modified in order to examine some specific areas of functioning more directly or in greater detail than before. These included performance over a sustained period of time and impulsivity. The measures of verbal competence were also supplemented.

The specific changes made were as follows:
1. The four subtests of the Wechsler Intelligence Scale for Children, the Passage Recall and the Manual Dexterity tasks were retained. A different news story was used in the Passage Recall task.

2. The automated Symbol Digit Coding Task was extended so that it comprised 225 items instead of 45 and lasted on average for 7.5 instead of 1.5 minutes.

3. The Speed of Information Processing, Visual Perceptual Analysis Reaction Time, Finger Tapping and Trail-Making tasks and the assessment of vibration perception thresholds were omitted.

4. The British Picture Vocabulary Test (Dunn, Dunn, Whetton and Pintile, 1982), the Matching Familiar Figures Test (Kagan, Rosman, Day, Albert and Phillips, 1964) and the Spiral Maze Test (Gibson, 1977) were added to the test battery. Description of these three new tests are given in Appendix C.

2.9 Statistical Methods

The statistical significance of the differences between cases and controls on categorical variables was examined by means of chi-squared tests; differences between cases and controls on continuous measures were examined using t-tests for matched samples. The effect of frequency of solvent abuse and other multi-level factors relating to history of solvent abuse were examined by means of analyses of variance. Where appropriate, further details of the statistical methods used for particular sets of analyses are provided in the relevant parts of the Results section.

3 Results

3.1 Epidemiological Aspects of Solvent Abuse

As described earlier, although the screening questionnaire was administered in 16 schools in three boroughs, there were differences between the boroughs in the way schools were selected for participation in the study. The 13 schools in boroughs A and B were selected at random by the research team, but it was not possible to select the schools in borough C in this way. They were instead selected by the borough Education Department. In view of the possibility that the schools in borough C may have been preferentially selected because they had a reputation for high rates of drug and solvent abuse, the data from the schools in boroughs A and B provide a more unbiased estimate of the prevalence and pattern of solvent abuse. For this reason, the epidemiological findings reported here are based on the data obtained from the schools in these two boroughs.

3.1.1 Prevalence of Reported Solvent Abuse

Completed questionnaires were obtained from 4225 pupils attending the 13 schools in boroughs A and B. 251 (5.9%) of them answered "yes" to the question "Have you ever sniffed glue, solvents (or anything else) on purpose?". In addition, there were 45 (1.1%) who did not answer "yes" to this question, but who responded to the other questions on solvent abuse in a way which was judged to indicate that they might also have sniffed. Altogether, 3929 (93.0%) clearly denied having sniffed solvents.

Of the 251 children who acknowledged having sniffed, 151 (3.6% of the total sample) indicated that they had "sniffed enough to feel high or intoxicated", 26 (0.6%) did not know whether they had been intoxicated and the remaining 74 (1.7%) denied intoxication. The term 'solvent abuse' will henceforth be used to denote the practice of sniffing volatile substances *to the point of intoxication.*

3.1.2 Factors Affecting the Prevalence of Solvent Abuse
3.1.2.1 School
The prevalence of solvent abuse differed from school to school, ranging from less than 1% to more than 6%. Table 6 shows the prevalence among boys and girls in single-sex and coeducational schools. The rate was highest in the four girls' schools, lowest in the three boys' schools and intermediate in the six coeducational schools. However, when boys and girls attending the same schools are compared, no important differences in rates of solvent abuse were observed.

3.1.2.2 School Year and Sex
Table 7 shows the prevalence of solvent abuse among children attending coeducational schools broken down by school year and sex. The peak prevalence rate was the same in boys and girls (5.2%), but in girls it was observed among fourth year pupils (aged 14 to 15 years), whereas in boys it was observed in fifth year pupils (aged 15 to 16 years).

Expressing these findings in a different way, in 13 to 14 year old pupils the rate was somewhat lower in boys than in girls (1.7% vs 3.3%), whereas no major differences were observed in 14-15 year olds (5.0% vs 5.2%), and among 15 to 16 year olds the rate was higher in boys than in girls (5.3% vs 3.3%).

3.1.3 Frequency of Solvent Abuse

Tables 8 and 9 show the reported frequency of solvent abuse in questionnaire-identtified cases, broken down by school year (Table 8) and sex (Table 9). In each school year and in both sexes, approximately half of them had sniffed only once or twice. At the other end of the frequency distribution, about one in 13 had abused solvents more than 30 times. The distribution of frequencies of abuse is similar among boys and girls, although there is a suggestion in the data that boys may be more likely than girls to abuse solvents frequently (an indication also noted in the findings of the pilot studies).

3.1.4 Types of Products Abused

The types of product that had been abused are shown in Tables 10 and 11 together with the number of children who acknowledged having abused them on the questionnaire. The total exceeds the number of cases because many children had abused more than one different product. Typewriter correction fluids were the most popular product and had been abused by nearly two-thirds of the cases. Butane gas and glue had been abused by about a third of the sample. Dry cleaning and degreasing agents, petrol, amyl (or butyl) nitrite, paints and aerosols had also been abused, but in each case by less than 5% of the solvent abusers, and taken together by about 15%. Nearly half of the boys who had abused solvents had sniffed glue, in contrast to only about one in six of the girls (chi square = 16.70, 1 degree of freedom: $p<.001$). the boys were also significantly more likely than the girls to have abused petrol (Fisher's exact test: $p<0.05$). Typewriter correction fluids and amyl (or butyl) nitrite were slightly more likely to have been abused by the girls.

3.1.5 Number of Different Products Abused

Slightly more than half of the solvent abusers had abused only one product (see Tables 12 and 13). There was a significant difference between the sexes with respect to the number of products that had been abused. The boys were more likely than the girls to have tried three or more different products (chi square = 10.1, 1 df: $p < 0.0015$).

3.2 Comparison Between the Questionnaire, Interview and Toxicological Findings

3.2.1 Agreement Between the Questionnaire and Interview Findings

Table 14 shows the correspondence between the questionnaire and interview findings on the items concerned with whether or not the child had sniffed solvents to the point of intoxication. Of the 133 children who were positive on the self-completed questionnaire, solvent abuse was confirmed at interview in 106 (79.9%) cases. All of the 113 negative respondents confirmed at interview that they had not abused solvents.

3.2.2 Toxicological Findings of the Interview-confirmed Cases and Controls

It was not possible to conduct toxicological examinations on five of the 106 interview-confirmed cases and six of the 113 interview-confirmed controls. Among those who were toxicologically examined, seven of the 101 interview-confirmed cases (6.9%) and one of the 107 interview-confirmed controls were positive for volatile substances. Details of those who were positive on toxicological examination are shown in Table 15. In all of the cases, the substances identified were consistent with the product which was reported to have been abused most recently (1,1,1-trichloroethane in six cases who had last abused typewriter correction fluids, toluene in the remaining case who had most recently abused petrol). The control was positive for toluene for reasons which could not be satisfactorily explained.

Table 16 shows the relationship between the results of the toxicological examination and the length of time since solvents were last abused (as reported at interview). Generally speaking, the breath test was more likely to be positive among those cases who reported that they had abused solvents recently. Thus 40% of the cases (two of five) who acknowledged solvent abuse during the three days prior to assessment were positive on the breath test, whereas only 3.7% (three of eighty) of those who had last abused solvents more than a month before the assessment were definitely positive. However, these results also make it clear that in the present study the toxicological examination could not be relied upon to detect all cases, or even a majority of cases, of recent solvent abuse.

3.3 The History and Pattern of Solvent Abuse in Cases Confirmed at Interview

The cases who were interviewed formed a selected sample. They were selected from those who gave a positive response on the questionnaire, but selection was weighted towards the upper end of the frequency of abuse distribution. Table 17 compares the frequency of solvent abuse among the interview-confirmed cases and the positive questionnaire respondents from boroughs A, B and C. For comparative purposes, the Table also shows the frequency among positive questionnaire respondents from boroughs A and B. The inclusion of the three schools from borough C had little effect on the distribution of frequencies of solvent abuse among positive questionnaire respondents. However, the proportion of cases who had sniffed more than 30 times was approximately twice as high in the interview-confirmed cases than among the positive questionnaire respondents.

These three groups were also compared to see whether there were any other differences between the interview-confirmed cases and the positive questionnaire respondents in their pattern of solvent abuse. None were found. As shown in Tables 18 and 19, the three groups were comparable with respect to the type and number of different products abused. (For the sake of brevity, the interview-confirmed cases will from now on be referred to simply as 'the cases').

As described earlier, the interview included some additional questions about the child's history and practice of solvent abuse which were not asked on the self-completed screening questionnaire. Table 20 shows when the cases had first sniffed solvents and how recently they had done so. Just over half of them had first sniffed during the 12 months preceding the interview and a similar proportion had last sniffed during the preceding six months. Eight of the 103 cases on whom data were obtained had sniffed during the week prior to interview.

Data on the social context and preferred place for sniffing were obtained only from those who had sniffed at least five times. These data are presented in Table 21. For the majority of the cases, sniffing was always a group activity engaged in with other sniffers, but for a substantial minority (21.3%) sniffing was at least sometimes a solitary act. Most of the cases usually sniffed in public spaces such as cemeteries, parks, streets or on patches of waste land, a few usually sniffed at their own or at friends' homes and two said that they usually sniffed at school.

3.4 Background Characteristics of the Solvent Abusers

3.4.1 Age, Sex and Ethnic Background
Table 22 compares the age, sex and ethnic background of the cases and controls. The two groups were matched for school year as well as sex and, not surprisingly, they were essentially similar in terms of age: the mean age of both groups was 15 years 0 months. There were, however, significant differences between the two groups in ethnic background. The cases were significantly *less* likely than the controls to be black. There were not many children of Indian or Pakistani ancestry in the study samples, but it appeared that they too might be underrepresented among the solvent abusers.

3.4.2 Family and Domestic Factors
As shown in Table 23, the domestic circumstances of the solvent abusers were generally less favourable than those of the controls. They were slightly less likely to be living with both their 'natural' parents, slightly more likely to come from

families living in rented accommodation, and significantly more likely to be members of large sibships than the controls. In addition, they were slightly less likely to come from homes in which the main breadwinner had a non-manual occupation, and significantly more likely to come from homes in which nobody was employed. Essentially the same pattern of associations emerged when cases and controls who were non-concordant for ethnic background were excluded from the comparison.

3.4.3 General Health and Accidents

Table 24 compares the cases and controls on a few indices of general health. The solvent abusers were 1.3 cm shorter than the controls. This difference was not statistically significant. There also were no significant differences between the two groups in terms of absences from school due to illness or whether or not they had taken prescribed medicines during the week prior to interview. The solvent abusers had received hospital treatment for accidents more often than the controls, but again these differences were not statistically significant (although see data in Table 41 on accidents reported at follow-up). Table 25 shows the accident data broken down by sex. Among both the solvent abusers and the controls, boys were more likely to report having had many accidents requiring hospital treatment, although this difference was statistically significant only among the controls.

3.4.4 Respiratory Health and Allergies

Table 26 presents the findings relating to the respiratory health of the cases and controls. The levels of self-reported asthma or wheeziness, and bronchitis or pneumonia during the past twelve months were high in both groups but there were no significant differences between them in terms of whether or not they had suffered from these complaints or whether they were currently using an aerosol inhaler for legitimate reasons. The results of the two groups on tests of lung function were also closely comparable. There were, however, significant differences between the questionnaire responses of the cases and controls to items concerned with coughing and shortness of breath: in each case the solvent abusers were much more likely to report these symptoms.

These last findings were reanalysed separately among current cigarette smokers and non-smokers to see whether the self-reported respiratory complaints of the solvent abusers could be explained in terms of the strong association between respiratory complaints and cigarette smoking. The results of these analyses were equivocal. In both smokers and non-smokers, coughing (especially first thing in the morning) was significantly more common among the solvent abusers than among the controls, suggesting that the association between solvent abuse and coughing could *not* be explained in terms of cigarette smoking. However, with shortness of breath, there was little difference between the solvent abusers and their controls after controlling for cigarette smoking status.

3.4.5 Cigarette Smoking

The solvent abusers were much more likely to smoke cigarettes than their controls. The figures shown in Table 27 come from the interview except where indicated, but the questionnaire findings were almost identical. Nearly a third of the controls, but only one of the 105 cases, claimed that they had never smoked a cigarette; and whereas 78% of the cases described themselves as current smokers, this was true of only 19% of the controls. The solvent abusers were also more likely to smoke frequently than the controls. Of those who smoked, 32% of the cases, but only 16% of the controls smoked more than ten cigarettes a day. However, perhaps the most striking difference between the two groups concerned how recently they had smoked. At interview 65% of the cases, but only 12.4% of the controls, said that they had smoked earlier that day (presumably on the way to school or during break). In addition, the mothers of the cases were significantly more likely to be smokers than the mothers of the controls.

3.4.6 Alcohol Consumption

The findings with respect to alcohol consumption (shown in Table 28) are similar to those for cigarette smoking, but the differences between the cases and controls, although statistically significant, are not quite as marked. Whereas 57% of the cases said at interview that they had drunk alcohol during the preceding week, only 34% of the controls had done so. As many as a third of the controls said that they drank only on special occasions such as parties or at Christmas, whereas less than 10% of the solvent abusers restricted their drinking to occasions of this kind.

Only five cases and one control admitted to getting drunk as often as once a week. It seems likely however that these estimates err on the side of sobriety: as many as 20 of the cases (25.0% of those who drank) and four of the controls (9.5% of those who drank) said that they had in fact been drunk during the week preceding the interview.

3.4.7 Behavioral and Emotional Aspects of Health

As described earlier, the self-completed questionnaire included a 15-item checklist which asked about various behavioral and emotional problems. Tables 29 and 30 show the number of cases and controls who indicated each problem as having occurred 'often' during the preceding 12 months. The figures for boys and girls are presented separately. On all of the comparisons but one; the problems were acknowledged more often by the cases than the controls. The items that significantly distinguished the boys who abused solvents from their controls were primarily those relating to anti-social conduct (poor concentration, involvement in fights, stealing, destructive behavior and truancy). The items that significantly distinguished the girls who abused solvents from their controls (not eating, stomach aches, poor concentration, worrying, truancy, misery and loneliness) reflected emotional disturbances more explicitly. Poor concentration and truancy were the only items that distinguished both the boys and the girls who abused solvents.

Responses to each of the checklist items were scored on a 0 to 3 scale (according to whether the behaviour was acknowledged as occurring 'Not at all', 'rarely', 'sometimes', or 'often'), and the scores were aggregated to produce an overall score for each child ranging from 0 to 45. The overall scores can be seen as providing a summary measure of the severity and extent of conduct and emotional problems. As shown at the foot of the Tables 29 and 30, in both sexes there were significant differences in mean overall scores between the solvent abusers and the controls.

In order to investigate whether there was anything *distinctive* about the pattern of problems acknowledged by the solvent abusers, it was necessary to compare their pattern of individual item responses with those of a control group with comparably high overall scores. Not many of the 105 individually assessed controls had high overall checklist scores, and so instead, new control groups were selected from the sample of more than 4000 pupils who had denied solvent abuse on the original screening questionnaire. Cut-off scores were empirically derived such that when pupils with scores falling below the cut-off point were excluded from the sample, the mean overall score of the controls was similar to that of the solvent abusers. In view of the sex difference in mean overall scores, separate cut-off scores were established for boys and girls. In order to equate the mean scores of the controls with those of the solvent abusers, it was necessary to exclude boys with overall scores of 13 or less and girls with overall scores of 16 or less.

Table 31 compares the individual item responses of the boys who abused solvents with those of the boys from the original questionnaire sample who had comparably high checklist scores. Table 32 presents the same comparison for the girls. In contrast to the results of the preceding analyses, the pattern of problems acknowledged by the solvent abusers was essentially the same in both boys and girls. In both sexes, the only items that the solvent abusers were at least twice as likely to acknowledge as the controls were those relating to misconduct: fighting, stealing, destructive behavior and truancy. The only exception to this pattern was for 'destructive behavior' among girls which did not emerge as a distinguishing item, possibly because the numbers involved were very small and the data are therefore likely to be less reliable.

3.4.8 School Attendance and Performance

In contrast to the self-report data on truancy, the information on school attendance collected from the school registers showed no significant difference between the cases and controls (see Table 33). There was, however, a significant difference between the two groups in the mean number of half days on which they had registered late: the solvent abusers were late more often than the controls.

At interview, the solvent abusers appraised their school performance as being 'not very good' significantly more often than the controls. They were also significantly less likely to enjoy good relations with their teachers. There was a tendency for more of the controls than the cases to prefer 'academic' subjects such as English and math, but this difference was not statistically significant.

3.5 Psychological Test Results

The battery of psychological measures used in the initial assessments consisted of 15 different tests, but on several of them, more than one measure of performance was recorded. Altogether, the battery provided 35 'main' measures which were used to examine the effects of solvent abuse on level of performance. Four of these were aggregate scores reflecting performance on combinations of other measures.

In addition to these 35 main psychological test variables, a subsidiary set of ten other measures was examined. The standard deviation of each subject's mean reaction time (RT) over several trials was calculated on each of the ten RT measures from the Visual Discrimination, Symbol-Digit Coding and Two-choice Reaction Time tasks. These ten subsidiary measures were included to test the secondary hypothesis that exposure to solvents results primarily in *variability* in behavior and performance rather than a decrease in the *level* of performance (cf. Knave, Olson, Elofsson et al, 1978).

The main set of variables was used routinely to examine the relationships between psychological test performance and the various aspects of the child's history of solvent abuse; the subsidiary set was used only for the basic comparison between cases and controls.

Twenty five of the 105 case-control pairs were non-concordant for ethnic background and these pairs were excluded from all of the analyses of the psychological test results. The analyses were therefore concerned with the remaining 80 case-control pairs who were matched for ethnic background (as well as school, school year and sex).

The cases and controls were compared by subtracting the score of each case from that of its matched control and performing t-tests to examine whether the mean difference scores differed significantly from zero. The effect of frequency of solvent abuse (and other multi-level factors relating to the child's history of solvent abuse) was examined by means of analyses of variance carried out on these mean difference scores to test the hypothesis that the subgroups differed significantly from each other.

Findings are reported as statistically significant if the results of significance tests indicated that the null hypothesis should be rejected at the 5% level of chance. However, it should be noted that in view of the large number of tests carried out, a few of the measures (two or three of the 45 variables that comprised the main and subsidiary sets) would be expected to show differences between groups at this level of significance, solely on the basis of chance. Rather than adopt a more stringent significance level (which might obscure a smaller, but consistently observed effect of solvent abuse), we considered it more informative to declare all differences observed at the 5% level of chance and take account of the number of significance tests carried out *after* reviewing the consistency of the pattern of psychological test findings.

3.5.1 Comparison Between Cases and Controls

Table 34 shows the psychological test scores of the two groups. The solvent abusers performed significantly less well than their matched controls on just four of the 35 main neuropsychological outcome measures. Three of these - vocabulary, prorated Verbal IQ and prorated Full Scale IQ - were from the Wechsler Scales. The fourth measure which showed a significant difference between groups was the 'inhibitory' version of the reaction time task, on which the solvent abusers failed to *withhold* inappropriate responses more often than the controls.

Breath samples were obtained immediately after psychological testing from 77 of these 80 cases, and in seven of them the toxicological examination showed solvent in the child's breath. In order to examine the possibility that the significant differences in psychological test performance reflect an *acute* effect of recent solvent abuse, the comparisons between the cases and controls were repeated after excluding these seven cases and their matched controls. When this was done, the four measures that had previously shown a significant difference between groups continued to do so.

In order to identify potentially confounding social factors that might have obscured other significant differences between groups, each of the six socio-demographic variables shown in Table 23 was examined in relation to the psychological test results of the cases and controls. Three of these variables - sibship size, parental socio-economic status and housing tenure - showed a relationship with psychological test performance that was considered strong enough, and sufficiently independent of the relationship with the other two, to warrant taking their effects into account.

Multiple regression analyses were performed to control for differences between groups on these three variables and on ethnic background. Sibship size, housing tenure and parental socio-economic status were categorised as indicated in Table 23. Ethnic background was dummy coded to allow classification of the various possible permutations of this variable (as shown in Table 22) in the cases and controls. Cases and controls who were not from the same school were excluded from the analysis. Only one of the thirty-five main measures showed a significant difference between cases and controls after taking into account the effects of these various confounding factors: the solvent abusers made significantly more left/right errors on the two-choice reaction time test ($t = 2.45$; $p = 0.040$).

Finally, Table 35 shows the scores of the cases and controls on the subsidiary set of psychological test variables (comprising the standard deviations of mean reaction time responses on ten different measures). Only one variable showed a significant difference between groups: the solvent abusers showed greater variability of reaction times when correctly using the right hand to respond on the inhibitory version of the two-choice RT task.

3.5.2 Relationship with Frequency of Solvent Abuse

Table 36 shows the relationship between frequency of solvent abuse and psychological test performance among the cases and controls matched for ethnic back ground. The scores shown are the mean of the case-control difference scores in each of the subgroups (positive scores indicate that the scores of the controls were higher than those of the cases, negative scores indicate the opposite pattern). There were no statistically significant differences between the five subgroups on any of the tests. In order to check the robustness of these findings with larger subsamples, the five subgroups were collapsed into three groups of roughly equal size (one to two times, three to nine times and ten or more times) and the above analyses were repeated. As before, there were no significant effects of frequency of solvent abuse on any of the test measures.

3.5.3 Relationship with Other Aspects of Solvent Abuse

The psychological test results of the cases and controls were examined in relation to (a) the length of time since the child's most recent episode of solvent abuse, (b) the type of product abused, (c) the number of different products abused, and (d) the length of time since solvents had first been abused. Table 37 summarizes the results of these analyses by indicating the tests on which statistically significant relationships were observed.

3.5.3.1 Most Recent Episode of Solvent Abuse

A statistically significant relationship was found between the time since the child had last abused solvent and psychological test performance on four measures - the block design subtest and prorated performance IQ of the WISC, the number of errors on the two-choice reaction time task and the speed of finger tapping with the right index finger.

Relative to their controls, the cases who had sniffed solvents during the week or month preceding assessment made *fewer* errors on the choice reaction time task than those who had last sniffed more than a month ago. On the test of right index finger tapping speed, no systematic relationship with recency of sniffing was discernible. On both the block design subtest and prorated Performance IQ, the subgroup that had sniffed during the week prior to assessment obtained *higher* scores than their controls, and the pattern of case-control differences across the five subgroups showed no obvious trend. Thus, on all four measures on which significant differences were found the relationship between recency of abuse and psychological test performance was either inconsistent or incoherent.

3.5.3.2 Type of Product Abused

Examination of the effects of different types of product was made difficult because, as shown in Table 19, approximately half of the cases had used more than one substance. Thus, although Table 18 shows that 80 of the interviewed cases had used typewriter correction fluids, and that 32 had used glue and 29 had used butane gas, the numbers who had used *only* these products, and who were matched with a control of the same ethnic background, were 35, 8 and 3, respectively. The numbers who had used products other than typewriter correction fluids were far too small to warrant statistical analysis of the findings and no significant differences were found between those who had abused *only* typewriter fluids and their controls.

38

3.5.3.3 Number of Different Products Abused

When the psychological test results were examined in relation to the number of different types of substances that the child had sniffed, a statistically significant effect on vibration sensation threshold measured at the ankle was found. The relationship appeared to be systematic, but in fact the direction of the effect was opposite to that predicted: cases who had abused the most products showed the lowest thresholds of vibration perception relative to their controls. None of the other thirty- four measures showed a statistically significant effect.

3.5.3.4 Time since First Abused Solvents

A statistically significant relationship was found between the time since the child had started to sniff and performance on four of the 35 measures. These were the number of errors on the simple version of the visual discrimination task, mean reaction time on the two-choice RT task, and the speed of finger tapping both with the right index finger and also when alternate taps with the right index and middle fingers were required. However, only with the first of these measures was there a coherent and systematic relationship, with progressively more errors being made, relative to the controls, the longer the time since the child had first sniffed.

3.6 Educational Test Results Antecedent to Solvent Abuse

Data on test performance *prior* to solvent abuse (obtained from the schools) came from either tests of reading ability or verbal reasoning tests. Satisfactory data were available from the files of 73 (69.5%) of the 105 cases and 83 (79.0%) of the 105 controls. As shown in Table 38, the distribution of types of test from which data were obtained was very similar in the two groups.

Table 39 compares the mean scores on these tests with those from equivalent tests administered at the initial assessment. The antecedent reading test scores are compared with scores on the reading test administered as part of the initial assessment; antecedent verbal reasoning test scores are compared with initial assessment Verbal IQ estimates. The data are presented separately for solvent abusers and controls matched for ethnic background.

Sample sizes are relatively small because the analyses are restricted to matched pairs for whom a score was available on both occasions. Comparisons are therefore between scores of the same subjects at two points in time.

On both the reading and verbal reasoning tests, the scores of the controls increased (by 3.1 points and 3.3 points respectively), whereas the scores of the solvent abusers decreased (by 2.8 points and 5.0 points respectively).

The statistical significance of these findings was examined by (a) calculating 'change-over-time' scores for each case and control, (b) subtracting the change score of each case from that of his or her control, and (c) performing paired t-tests on the resulting difference scores. The difference between groups in changes in reading test scores was not statistically significant (t [18 df] = - 1.26), but, relative to their controls, the solvent abusers appeared to show a significant deterioration in verbal reasoning test scores (t [20 df] = - 2.16).

3.7 Follow-up

3.7.1 The Follow-up Samples and Assessments

Figure 2 shows how the follow-up samples were composed. Of the 105 matched pairs who were initially assessed, 24 were fifth form pupils (aged 15 to 16 years) when first seen and, for reasons given earlier, no attempt was made to trace them. In addition, three cases and four controls from the remaining 81 matched pairs had been initially tested in 1983/4 or 1985/6 and scheduling difficulties made it impossible to attempt to trace them.

An attempt was made to trace the remaining 77 controls and 78 cases whose initial assessments had been carried out in 1984/5. Seventy two (93.5%) of these controls were found and tested at follow-up, whereas only 61 (78.2%) cases were found and retested. This difference is statistically significant (chi square = 7.5 with 1 df; p = 0.006). Of the 5 (6.5%) controls and 17 (21.8%) cases who could not be retested, one control and four cases had moved to a new school or had been transferred to a support unit (for difficult-to-manage pupils) attached to their old school. The remaining four controls and 13 cases were not retested because they were absent from school when the follow-up assessments were carried out. Fifteen of these 17 absentees were fifth year pupils.

At follow-up, one of the 72 controls reported that she had abused solvents for the first time during the interval between the two assessments. She was therefore excluded from the follow-up control group. The final follow-up samples therefore consisted of 61 children who had abused solvents at some time in the past and 71
controls who had never done so.

The follow-up assessments were carried out on average 296.6 days (9.6 months) after the initial assessments (292.2 days later for the controls and 301.8 days later for the cases). The mean interval between the initial and follow-up assessments was less than 12 months because, as described earlier, the follow-up assessments had to be condensed into the autumn and spring terms of 1985-6, rather than spread over the school year like the initial assessments.

3.7.2 Comparison Between Cases and Controls at Follow-up

The 61 cases and 71 controls who comprised the follow-up samples, included 57 of the original matched pairs, 4 cases whose matched control could not be retested and 14 controls whose matched case could not be retested. Rather than reduce the sample size further by excluding unmatched cases or controls who had already been retested, it was decided to analyse the follow-up data using statistical tests for unmatched pairs.

3.7.2.1 Age, School Year, Sex and Ethnic Background

Table 40 shows the age, school year, sex and ethnic background of the cases and controls who were found and examined at follow-up. The two groups were closely comparable in terms of mean age, school year and sex distribution. The mean age of both groups at follow-up was 15 years 6 months and 72% of each group were 5th year pupils (aged 15 to 16 years) with the remainder coming from the 4th year (aged 14 to 15 years). As with the initial assessment samples, approximately three- fifths of the children in each group were girls (62% of the solvent abusers and 59% of the controls). The underrepresentation of black children in the solvent abuse group noted at initial assessment was also still apparent although the difference was marginally less marked than before.

3.7.2.2 Accidents and Illnesses Since Initial Assessment

The children who were re-examined at follow-up were asked about their experience of accidents and illnesses during the interval between the two assessments and whether they were taking any prescribed medicines at the time of the follow-up examination. The findings are shown in Table 41. As before, there were no significant differences between the two groups in the likelihood of their having missed school because of illness, and again the proportion in each group who were taking prescribed medicines was similar. However, the solvent abusers were more than twice as likely than the controls (27.9% vs. 11.3%) to have had hospital treatment or an admission for an accident or illness. This difference is statistically significant ($t = 2.73$ with 72.3 df: $p = 0.012$) and would appear to reflect a greater likelihood of their having received hospital *treatment* following an accident: 16 (26.2%) of the solvent abusers had received hospital treatment following an accident in contrast to only 6 (8.4%) of the controls, and only one child in each group had been admitted following an accident.

3.7.2.3 Solvent Abuse Since Initial Assessment

The pattern of solvent abuse during the 9 month interval between the initial and follow-up assessments is shown in Tables 42 and 43. As mentioned earlier, one member of the control group abused solvents for the first time during this period and she was therefore excluded from the follow-up control group. As shown in Table 42, fifteen of the sixty-one (24.6%) who were traced and examined at follow-up indicated that they had continued to abuse solvents between the two assessments. The types of product that had been abused between the two assessments were much the same as those that were acknowledged by the full sample of cases at initial assessment: typewriter correction fluids had been used by roughly two thirds of them, glue and butane gas had each been used by about a third, while other products had been used by a smaller proportion of cases. Table 43 shows when the cases who were followed had last abused solvents. Comparison between these data and the corresponding data from the initial assessment (shown in Table 20) shows a general increase in the length of time since solvents had last been abused. Thus, 3.5% of the cases had abused solvents during the week preceding the follow-up assessments (compared with 7.8% during the week preceding the initial assessments) and 8.8% had abused solvents during the month preceding follow-up (compared with 18.5%). Conversely, 57.4% of the follow-up sample had abused solvents more than a year ago (compared with 24.3% of the initial assessment sample). These data indicate that, generally speaking, in the sample of cases identified in this study, solvent abuse was a more recent or current practice at initial assessment than it was at follow-up.

3.7.2.4   Illicit Drug Use (Ever)

At follow-up the opportunity was taken to supplement the data on the use of solvents, tobacco and alcohol by asking about the use of various types of illicit drug. The findings are shown in Table 44. As might be expected, a higher proportion of solvent abusers than controls had used each type of drug, and with cannabis and amphetamines the numbers were large enough to make the difference statistically significant. Cannabis was by far the most popular illicit drug and had
been used by more than three-quarters of the children who had abused solvents and roughly one in eight of the randomly selected controls. None of the other illicit drugs had been taken by any of the controls. A fifth of the solvent abusers acknowledged having taken amphetamines but less than 5% had taken cocaine, LSD or other "hard" drugs.

The number of children who had used cannabis and amphetamines was high enough to permit examination of the frequency and recency of their use in the two groups. Frequent cannabis smoking (defined as more than thirty times ever) was generally more common among the solvent abusers than among those of the controls who had smoked: as many as a third of the solvent abusers who had smoked cannabis had done so frequently, whereas none of the controls had used cannabis more often than thirty times. None of the children in either group had taken either drug earlier on the same day as the assessment, but three solvent abusers and one control had smoked cannabis the day before, and an additional nine solvent abusers and one control had smoked two or three days before the assessment. Thus, nearly 20% of the total sample of solvent abusers had smoked cannabis during the three days prior to assessment. Less than 3% of the total sample of controls had used cannabis as recently as this.

3.7.2.5 Psychological Test Results

As with the psychological test results, from the initial assessment, the findings at follow-up were analysed after excluding cases and controls who were non-concordant for ethnic background. This left 37 matched pairs. Their results on those tests that were readministered at follow-up are shown in Table 45; the findings on tests that were newly introduced at follow-up are shown in Table 46. On both sets of measures, there were no significant differences between groups.

4 Discussion

4.1 Epidemiological Aspects of Solvent Abuse

4.1.1 Overall Prevalence

4.1.1.1 Findings from this Study

In the two boroughs where schools were selected at random by the research team, 5.9% of those who completed the questionnaire indicated that they had sniffed solvents at some time in the past. However, a sizable minority of these cases either denied intoxication or were unsure whether they had been intoxicated. If only those who had "sniffed enough to feel high or intoxicated" are included, the rate becomes 3.6%.

Before comparing these estimates of the prevalence of solvent abuse with those obtained in other studies, it is important to consider the accuracy and validity of the methods of identifying adolescents who had abused solvents in the present investigation. Two sets of factors that might affect reported prevalence rates need to be considered. First, the effects of non-participation in the survey, due to absenteeism or parental refusal, need to be discussed. Second, the validity of the methods of identifying solvent abuse in those who did take part need to be taken into account.

15.8% of the target population were absent from school on the day the questionnaire was administered and, as in virtually all other drug questionnaire surveys, it was not feasible to trace this group in order to include them in the survey. However, four separate findings from the present study indicate that solvent abusers are likely to be overrepresented among these absentees. First, the self-report data from the questionnaire indicated that the solvent abusers rated themselves as much more likely than the controls to have been frequently absent from school without justification. Second, the school registers showed that the solvent abusers who were interviewed were absent from school more often than the controls: the difference was not statistically significant but the direction of the effect was consistent with the other evidence on absenteeism. Third, significantly more of the cases than the controls were absent from school when attempts were made to find them by the research team for the follow-up assessments. Fourth, the absentees *were* followed-up in the pilot studies conducted in two schools, and it was found that their rate solvent abuse was approximately three times higher than that of those present for the initial questionnaire survey. The conclusion that solvent abusers are overrepresented among school absentees is in agreement with Kandel's (1975) findings. To the extent that they are overrepresented among those not included in the survey, the prevalence figures are likely to underestimate the true prevalence.

Another group not included in the survey are those pupils whose parents refused permission for them to take part. Eleven percent of the target population were excluded for this reason, although as noted earlier, there was some overlap between this group and the absentees already discussed. Nothing is known about this group and there is little evidence from other studies about what effect their non-participation will have had on the prevalence estimates. It may be that the parents who refused permission for their children to take part are highly conscientious people who aim to exert control over the lives and activities of their children in many situations outside the home, a control which extends to their children's recreational pastimes. On the other hand, it is equally plausible that both they and their children are generally uncooperative and non-compliant in their dealings with schools and other outside agencies.

With those children who took part in the survey and who completed the questionnaire, other possible sources of error have to be considered. First, there is the issue of false negatives. It seems very likely that a number of children who had in fact abused solvents denied having done so on the questionnaire. Various steps were taken to minimize the size of this group. Full scale pilot studies were conducted in four different schools in order to improve the wording of the questionnaire and the procedures used in administering it. An attempt was made to minimize the impact of the questions on solvents by embedding them among other items concerned with general and respiratory health. The children were told not to record their names on the questionnaire and the confidentiality of the survey was emphasized in a variety of ways. Nevertheless, it would be unrealistic to imagine that the questionnaire was successful in identifying *all* children who had abused solvents. The interview findings of the children who denied solvent abuse on the questionnaire provide some reassurance about false negative responses: none of the 113 possible controls acknowledged solvent abuse at interview. However, it needs to be acknowledged that a child who falsely denies solvent abuse on an anonymous questionnaire is unlikely to admit it during a short face-to-face research interview, whatever the skills of the interviewer. It would seem reasonable to conclude that the questionnaire may have missed some children who had abused solvents, leading to an underestimate in prevalence, but the magnitude of this underestimation is unknown.

Second, the issue of false positives has to be considered. Roughly one in five of those who acknowledged solvent abuse on the questionnaire subsequently denied the practice during the face-to-face interview. If only the interview-confirmed cases are accepted as valid, the overall prevalence of solvent abuse in this study falls from 3.6% to 2.8%. However, although it was hoped at the outset that the interview would provide a more valid assessment of the child's history of solvent abuse, there is no absolute way of determining whether this was the case. Certainly, the interview was essential in identifying a handful of children who had given frivolous positive answers on the questionnaire, but with many of the others it is possible that the positive response to the anonymous questionnaire had been truthful and the child was just reluctant to admit having abused solvents at face-to-face interview. Whether or not these children should be counted as cases depends on whether it is more important to avoid false positives or false negatives. In examining the neuropsychological consequences of solvent abuse, we regarded the former as more important. Positive respondents on the screening questionnaire who subsequently denied solvent abuse at interview were therefore excluded from the group of cases, however implausible their denial may have seemed. However, in examining the prevalence of solvent abuse, we regarded this definition of a case as too stringent as it would have excluded some adolescents whom we thought, on balance, probably had abused solvents. The prevalence findings discussed below are therefore based on the data from the self-completed questionnaire and no correction has been made to the rates to take into account the number of cases who denied solvent abuse at interview. An additional advantage of this approach is that it facilitates direct comparisons with the results of other questionnaire surveys.

In summary, therefore, 5.9% of the questionnaire respondents in randomly selected schools acknowledged having sniffed solvents at some time in the past. This figure falls to 3.6% if only those who indicated that they had sniffed to the point of intoxication are included. However, these figures are likely to underestimate the true prevalence by an unknown amount because, as in all other published studies, they do not take false negatives into account and they neglect the higher rate of solvent abuse among absentees.

4.1.1.2 Comparability with Findings of Other Prevalence Studies
A large number of other surveys have provided data on the prevalence of solvent abuse in secondary school children. They have varied greatly in size, scope and quality, as well as in the findings they have yielded. Table 47 summarizes the overall prevalence rates from a number of different surveys conducted in the UK and elsewhere in the world. Overall prevalence rates ranging from 2% to more than 50% have been reported.

Before considering the possible reasons for the huge differences in reported rates, it is important to recognize that there is no good reason for expecting prevalence rates to be uniform across studies. Solvent abuse is a behavior that by all accounts is subject to fad and fashion among teenagers. Like many other teenage activities (eg, skate-boarding), it is markedly subject to peer group influences (Merrill, 1985) and, for most of those involved, enthusiasm for the practice does not last long (see below). In behavior, if not in etiology, it appears to conform reasonably well to an epidemic model of acute infectious illnesses, and rapid changes over time in the number of people involved *within* a given population are to be expected. Accordingly, differences in rates *between* populations will tend to be relatively unstable.

Nevertheless, there are also several artifacts that contribute to the variability in reported prevalence rates. First, there are differences between studies in the age range of the populations studied. As discussed in greater detail below, prevalence rates have been found to vary markedly according to the age group under consideration, and for this reason it is necessary to look at age-specific rates, rather than overall rates, when comparing the findings of different studies.

Second, although most studies have presented estimates of the prevalence of solvent abuse *at any time in the past*("ever"), some, notably the Canadian studies of Smart and his colleagues, have presented the rates in terms of the proportion who have sniffed recently (eg, "within the past six months"). Obviously, whether or not solvent abuse is linked to a particular time frame will affect prevalence rates. In the present study, for example, only about half of those who had ever abused solvents had done so during the preceding six months.

Third, there are major differences between studies in the wording of the questions on sniffing, particularly in terms of whether or not reference has been made to the experience of intoxication. The important surveys conducted by Smart, Adlaf and Goodstadt (1985) in Ontario and by Johnston, Bachman and O'Malley (1984) in the USA have asked about sniffing solvents "in order to get high". Similarly, in Plant et al's (1985) Edinburgh survey the questionnaire asked about trying various substances "either from curiosity or for kicks". By contrast, in Dunoon and Homel's (1984) New South Wales survey, the children were simply asked "How may times have you deliberately sniffed from spray cans or sniffed solvents like glue, petrol, thinners etc?" More than 50% of the questionnaire respondents indicated that they had sniffed, and the authors suggest that some of these cases may have done so completely innocently. In the present study, approximately 40% of those who acknowledged sniffing denied that (or were unsure whether) they had achieved intoxication, and when cases of this type were interviewed during the pilot studies, it appeared that most of them meant that they had simply smelled the substance in question without any thought of using it to get intoxicated. Many of the other studies listed in Table 47 have not reported the wording of the questions about solvents and it is therefore uncertain whether cases of this type are likely to have been included in the prevalence estimates.

Fourth, the prevalence estimates are likely to be affected by the way in which the questionnaire is presented and administered, and the extent to which the children who take part can be reassured about the confidentiality of their answers. It is difficult to assess the effect of factors of this kind in different studies partly because reports vary greatly in the amount of detail they provide about the procedural aspects of questionnaire administration, and partly because, where detail is provided, the effects of particular procedural variations are unknown. For example, although all surveys have been anonymous in the sense that the child was not required to write his or her name on the questionnaire, in some studies the questionnaire has been introduced, explained, supervised and collected by external field-workers, while in others this has been done by the school teachers (eg, Gossett, Lewis and Phillips, 1971) or the pupils themselves (eg, Porter, Vieira, Kaplan, Heesch and Colyar, 1973). With a socially disapproved activity such as solvent abuse, the effects of these procedural variants on the likelihood of obtaining false negative or false positive questionnaire responses could be substantial.

4.1.2 Variation by School Year

A peak in the prevalence of solvent abuse was observed among 4th year pupils (aged 14-15 years). This finding is consistent with the results of other population-based surveys (eg, Whitehead, 1970; Porter et al, 1973; Gossett et al, 1971), 14 year old age group in some parts of the world (eg, Smart et al, 1985). The peak in the age-specific prevalence of solvent abuse in the present study coincides the peak in the age distribution of deaths associated with solvent abuse in the UK (Anderson et al, 1985).

When age-specific prevalence rates were examined separately in the two sexes, it was observed that the peak rate occurred a year earlier in girls than in boys. Other surveys have not always presented their findings in a directly comparable way, but the data from the surveys conducted by Johnson, Donnelly, Scheble, Wein and Weitman (1971) and Whitehead (1970) also indicate that girls tend to abuse solvents at a slightly younger age than boys.

One of the most consistent findings in research on the use of drugs among secondary school children is the observation that solvent abuse occurs at a younger age than other forms of illicit substance abuse (eg, Whitehead, 1970; Gossett et al, 1971; Porter et al, 1973; Smart and Fejer, 1975; Castro and Valencia, 1980). As has been pointed out by others, the relatively low cost of products suitable for sniffing no doubt contributes to their popularity with younger, economically dependent adolescents. An additional factor that presumably also contributes arises from the fact that they can be purchased over the counter legitimately. They can therefore be bought in supermarkets by youngsters who have not yet developed the more complex social skills that are needed to negotiate the purchase of illicit drugs on the black market.

4.1.3 Variation by Sex

There were no important sex differences in the prevalence of solvent abuse when boys and girls attending the same schools were compared. Other population-based surveys have tended to indicate a somewhat higher rate in boys than in girls. Plant, Peck and Stuart (1984) and Plant et al (1985), for example, in their survey of school leavers in Edinburgh, found that 5.4% of boys and 4.0% of girls had abused solvents at some time in the past, and sex differences of a similar magnitude have been reported by others (eg, Whitehead, 1970; Kandel, Single and Kessler, 1976; Smart et al, 1985). The reasons for not finding a sex difference in the present study are unclear.

The sex differences found in these and other population-based studies of solvent abuse are not nearly as marked as those found in studies of fatalities or groups of solvent abusers attending clinics. For example, 88% of Bass' (1970) 'sudden sniffing deaths' were male, and in Anderson et al's (1985) national study of fatalities due to solvent abuse, males accounted for 95% of the sample. In Watson's (1978) series of consecutive referrals to a special clinic for solvent abusers in Glasgow 92% were male.

There are several possible factors that might explain the large differences between the findings of these studies (where the male preponderance has been very large) and the population-based studies (in which it has usually been slight). Firstly, boys might abuse solvents more frequently than girls. Solvent abusers who are referred to clinics tend to be chronic sniffers and if boys are more likely than girls to be chronic sniffers, a large sex difference in clinical referrals would be expected. The present study provides some limited support for this possibility inasmuch as the proportion of boys who had sniffed more than thirty times was more than twice as high as the proportion of girls who had done so. A second possibility is that boys might sniff solvents that are more lethal than those that girls sniff and this might account for the preponderance of boys among fatalities. This possibility is difficult to evaluate because little is known about the lethality of different volatile substances. It has been suggested that aerosols are particularly dangerous (Cohen, 1979) because of the risk of bronchospasm and laryngospasm when aerosols are sprayed directly into the mouth. It is of interest that in the present study the three cases who abused aerosols were all boys, but it seems unlikely that differences of this type and magnitude will account for the large sex differences in fatalities. Third, boys might sniff solvents in higher doses or for more prolonged periods than girls. The present study does not contribute toward the evaluation of this possibility. Fourth, boys who abuse solvents might be more likely than girls to get involved in accidents which bring them to the attention of hospital clinics or the county coroner. In keeping with this possibility, boys reported more accidents requiring hospital treatment than girls in the present study. The difference between the sexes was statistically significant only among the controls, but a similar trend was also apparent among the solvent abusers.

4.2 The Practice of Solvent Abuse

4.2.1 Pattern, History and Degree of Involvement in the Practice

The present study also provided information about the pattern and intensity of solvent abuse in secondary school children. In considering the findings and their mplications, it is important to bear in mind that the data come from three different sources. Data on the frequency, type and number of products that had been abused come from the self-completed questionnaire and the findings may therefore be regarded as representative of those who took part in the survey. Information on the duration of the practice (when it started and when solvents had last been sniffed) and information on the social context and preferred place of sniffing (whether it was generally pursued with others or alone and where it was done) was obtained at the initial interview.

The selection of cases for detailed assessment was intentionally biased toward the inclusion of those who had abused solvents more frequently, although, as far as could be ascertained, the cases identified by questionnaire and those confirmed at interview appeared to be closely comparable on other sniffing variables. Nevertheless, the possibility that the findings from the interview-confirmed cases reflect a somewhat heavier pattern of abuse than that which obtained in the general population needs to be kept in mind. Finally, information on the persistence of solvent abuse over the nine months following the initial interview comes from the sample of cases who were traced and examined at follow-up.

Generally speaking, the pattern of solvent abuse found in the questionnaire survey from the present study could best be described as primarily experimental. Nearly half of those who had abused solvents had done so only once or twice, and nearly four-fifths of them had sniffed fewer than ten times. At the other end of the frequency distribution, only 7.9% of them, or approximately one in thirteen, had sniffed more than thirty times. Finer gradation of the frequency of sniffing in this latter group was not possible because many of them found it very difficult to estimate just how often they had sniffed. The conclusion that frequent solvent abuse is relatively uncommon in unselected samples of secondary school attenders and that in most cases the practice is limited to a few experimental trials is generally consistent with the findings of other population-based studies. Kandel et al (1976), for example, found that 58% of New York State high school students who had used inhalants had done so only once or twice. Similar proportions of 'once or twice users' are also evident in the data from two surveys of nationally representative samples conducted in the USA (Abelson, Fishbourne and Cisin, 1977; Johnston, Bachman and O'Malley, 1984).

Typewriter correction fluids were the most popular products of abuse in the present study. They had been used by approximately two-thirds of the solvent abusers. Various glues and butane gas had each been abused by a third of this group. Other substances such as dry-cleaning fluids, petrol, amyl nitrite, paints and aerosols had also been tried by a few children, but in each case by less than 5% of the cases. Many other population-based surveys of solvent abuse have not reported systematic data on the types of products and comparisons are therefore difficult to make. However, the surveys of local secondary school children carried out by Lynch (1984) in Berkshire, Stuart (1985) in Macclesfield, Faber (1985) in East Sussex, and Pritchard et al (1986) in Bournemouth all indicate that glue was the most popular product of abuse. A few of the children in the present study mentioned at interview that glue used to be the most popular product. It seems likely that the popularity of different products will, like many other teenage preferences and pursuits, be subject to swings in fashion. Availability and accessibility probably also have a marked influence on the range of products abused. For example, Smart (1986) has pointed out that in American Indian communities where petrol sniffing is widespread, the petrol is often left in drums outside houses or in open dumps. The price of different products will also presumably have some effect on their popularity. It is difficult to assess the effect of efforts to restrict accessibility in the present survey, but casual inspection of local shops and supermarkets suggested that special precautions had sometimes been taken to restrict customer access to cans of glue and butane gas while bottles of typewriter correction fluid were usually more readily accessible for purchase or theft.

Half of the interview-confirmed cases could be described as 'current sniffers' (inasmuch as they had abused solvents within the six months period preceding the interview). Many had not been abusing solvents for long: more than 80% had first sniffed during the two years preceding the study and just over half had first sniffed during the preceding 12 months. It also seems that for many of them the practice is a transient one. More than three quarters of those who were traced and examined at follow-up had not sniffed during the nine month interval between the two assessments.

Although a substantial minority (21.2%) of the interview-confirmed cases said at interview that they had *sometimes* sniffed alone, for the majority of cases sniffing was always done with at least one other person. Zur and Yule (1990 b) found that solvent abuse in chronic cases was more likely to be a solitary act among those who sniffed most frequently. The fact that sniffing tended to be a social or group activity among the cases in the present study is consistent with their generally less intense and more experimental involvement in the practice.

4.2.2 Associations with Cigarette Smoking, Drinking and Illicit Drug Use

Like the data on the practice of solvent abuse, the data on cigarette smoking, alcohol consumption and use of illicit drugs also come from different sources. Questions on cigarette smoking and drinking were included in the initial and follow-up questionnaires. In addition, in order to provide a check on the validity of the child's questionnaire responses, similar questions on smoking and drinking were also asked at the initial interview. Agreement between initial questionnaire and interview responses to these questions was generally very good. Questions on illicit drug use were only included on the follow-up questionnaire, and the data on the use of these substances therefore come from the cases and controls who were traced and examined at follow-up.

There were very marked differences between the solvent abusers and the controls in their use of cigarettes, alcohol and illicit drugs. Generally speaking, not only were all classes of drug more likely to have been used, but they were more likely to have been used frequently and recently. The differences with respect to cigarette and cannabis smoking were particularly marked. Whether this indicates a general preference among solvent abusers for drugs that are inhaled, as opposed to ingested or injected, is uncertain. Alcohol differs from these inhaled substances not just in terms of method of consumption but currently also in terms of social acceptability, and it is possible that the high rates of cannabis use among the solvent abusers reflect a general preference for illicit substances. The number of children who had used other types of illicit drug was too low to allow a choice between these alternative explanations. None of the controls had used other illicit drugs and only a handful of the solvent abusers had tried LSD, cocaine or other 'hard' drugs.

4.3 Characteristics of Children Who Abused Solvents

4.3.1 Ethnic Background

There were significantly fewer black children in the sample of solvent abusers than among the randomly selected controls. A similar underrepresentation of blacks among solvent abusers was noted in studies comparing delinquent sniffers and non-sniffers carried out in South London (Dendle, unpublished) and Chicago (Sterling, 1964). Consistent with these findings from case-control studies, the prevalence of solvent abuse among children attending schools in New York State has also been found to be substantially lower among blacks than among whites (Kandel et al, 1976).

Most of the evidence relating to solvent abuse in other ethnic groups has come from North American studies. Early case series of children arrested for glue or solvent sniffing included a disproportionate number of youngsters of Spanish-American background (Glaser and Massengale, 1962) and the impression that 'Hispanics' are overrepresented in samples of solvent abusers has subsequently been confirmed in controlled studies comparing delinquents with and without a history of chronic solvent abuse (Barker and Adams, 1963; Sterling, 1964; Reed and May, 1984). Perez, Padilla, Ramirez, Ramirez and Rodriguez (1980) have linked the high frequency of solvent and psychoactive drug abuse among Mexican-American adolescents living on the outskirts of Los Angeles to the stresses of adapting from one culture to another.

The prevalence or solvent abuse also seems to be higher among American Indians, particularly those living in isolated village communities or reservations (Beauvais, Oetting and Edwards, 1985a and b). Kaufman (1973), for example, found that 62% of adolescents in a Pueblo Indian village in New Mexico had sniffed petrol, and Boeckx, Postl and Coodin (1977), on the basis of a two month stay in an isolated Indian reservation in north-eastern Manitoba, formed the impression that 'virtually all' of the 340 children and adolescents living there had sniffed petrol at one time or another, and nearly half of them had done so during the preceding three months. The high rates among American Indians do not appear to be restricted to petrol-sniffing or even solvent abuse in general, but are also observed for other drugs such as alcohol and marijuana (Oetting, Edwards, Goldstein and Garcia-Mason, 1980; Beauvais et al, 1985b). However, it is important to note that the rates in American Indians vary very much from group to group, with the highest rates tending to occur in groups with loosely organized social structures and weak tribal identities and in those whose culture and economy have been destroyed or undermined by rapid social change (May, 1982). Nurcombe, Bianchi, Money and Cawte (1970) have described a similar phenomenon in the Murngin people, a group of Aboriginal clans living on the Arnhem Land Reserve in Northern Australia.

4.3.2 Socio-economic and Domestic Circumstances

Many of the early US studies of solvent abusers noted an excess of children from large and divided families of low socio-economic status, often living in extremely impoverished circumstances (eg, Glaser and Massengale, 1962; Nylander, 1962; Barker and Adams, 1963; Sokol and Robinson, 1963; Massengale et al, 1963; Brozovsky and Winkler, 1965). The findings of the present study indicating that solvent abuse was associated with adverse background domestic circumstances are consistent with these previous reports, although the level of adversity encountered in the present sample was not nearly as dire as that described in many of the early reports. For example, whereas approximately 40% of the solvent abusers in the present study were not living with both their 'natural' parents, the proportion of cases coming from 'broken homes' was 57% in Brozovsky and Winkler's (1965) sample, 70% among Nylander's (1962) cases and 75% in the group referred to Massengale and his colleagues (1963).

It seems likely that the much stronger associations with social disadvantage found in many previous studies are due in part to the fact that the solvent abusers in all of the early studies cited above had either been apprehended by the police or referred for psychiatric treatment (or both). Such cases are more likely to come from disorganised and disadvantaged homes. By contrast, the sample in the present study was unselected for psychiatric or forensic history.

An additional but related factor concerns the frequency of solvent abuse in referred and unselected samples. Generally speaking, studies of clinic referrals are more likely to include a higher proportion of frequent or habitual solvent abusers than general population studies. The fact that the association between solvent abuse and background social disadvantage appeared to be weaker in the present study than in most studies of clinic referrals may be regarded as a reflection of the infrequency of habitual solvent abuse in the present sample.

Only a very limited amount of population-based research has been carried out to examine the social background characteristics of solvent abusers. Most of this work has concentrated on parental occupational status, and usually only relatively weak associations have been reported. Castro and Valencia (1980), for example, found that although the highest rates of solvent abuse in Mexico City were among children attending schools in areas of low socio-economic status (SES), the rates in the other areas did not show a consistent SES gradient. Gossett et al (1971), in a 1969 survey of over 56,000 Dallas high school students found that although most types of drugs were used more commonly in schools serving relatively affluent neighbourhoods, glue-sniffing was unrelated to the socio-economic reputation of the area. A similar pattern of findings comes from studies that have examined the SES of the household rather than the school neighborhood. In two recent British surveys, no association was found between parental occupational status and the prevalence of glue sniffing (NOP, 1982) or the use of illicit substances such as solvents (Plant et al, 1985).

4.3.3 General and Respiratory Health

The assessment of general health in the present study was not comprehensive, but instead was intended to focus on particular aspects of health implicated in clinical reports of chronic solvent abusers.

There were no significant differences between the solvent abusers and their controls in terms of current or recent illnesses, and generally speaking, the only evidence from the study that school children who abuse solvents suffer from worse physical health than others was their significantly greater likelihood of acknowledging coughing or shortness of breath on the self-completed questionnaire. This finding, however, might equally well be due to the fact that they were four times more likely than the controls to be current cigarette smokers. Separate analyses of the risk of respiratory complaints among current cigarette smokers and non-smokers suggested that although shortness of breath could be adequately explained in terms of cigarette smoking, the solvent abusers were more likely to complain of coughing than the controls even when the groups were equated for smoking status. Lung function tests, however, showed no significant differences between groups, a result consistent with the findings of Schikler et al (1984).

There were significant differences between the two groups in their experience of accidents. The solvent abusers reported more accidents requiring hospital treatment during the interval between the initial and follow-up assessments. This finding is consistent with the idea that adolescents who take drugs tend to lead lives in which danger and risk-taking play a generally more prominent role than usual (Jessor and Jessor, 1977).

Finally, there was no significant difference in mean height between the solvent abusers and their controls. This finding conflicts with the claim of Sokol and Robinson (1963) that children who abuse solvents tend to be of relatively short stature.

4.3.4 Behavioral and Emotional Problems

Although the idea that solvent abuse might be associated with psychological distress or disturbance is implicit in many studies, it is remarkable how infrequently this issue has been systematically examined. Early investigations tended to concentrate on the behavioral manifestations of acute intoxication, and since most of the cases were boys who had been arrested by the police for criminal or disorderly conduct while under the influence of glue, a relationship between glue sniffing and delinquency was quickly recognized. Subsequent enquiry often revealed a catalogue of other misdeeds.

Most of the studies carried out since then have been concerned with cases referred for psychological or psychiatric evaluation and treatment. The finding of high rates of psychiatric morbidity in these groups has not been entirely surprising.

In the present study, the sample of solvent abusers was unselected, but even so they were much more likely to indicate psychological problems than the controls. Virtually all of the items on the behavioral and emotional problems checklist were acknowledged as being a frequent problem more often by the solvent abusers, and, at interview, they were more likely to report difficulties in getting on with their teachers. They were also more likely to be registered as late in arriving for school, and as discussed earlier, they were more likely to be absent from school without justification.

There was a difference between the boys and the girls in the pattern of problems acknowledged on the checklist. The items that distinguished the boys who abused solvents from their controls (poor concentration, involvement in fights, stealing, destructive behaviour and truancy) were essentially those concerned with anti-social conduct, whereas those that distinguished the girls from their controls (not eating, stomach aches, poor concentration, worrying, truancy, misery and loneliness) reflected emotional problems more explicitly.

These findings are based solely on questionnaire self-report data. Undoubtedly it would have been an advantage if comparable data could have been obtained from the youngsters' parents and/or teachers, but the requirements of confidentiality put this out of the question. In any event, the desirability of 'objective' data has to be viewed in the light of who is best placed to identify the problem in question.

Parents are sometimes unaware of their adolescent child's misery and distress (Rutter, Graham, Chadwick and Yule, 1976) and secondary school teachers are unlikely to know much about their pupils' sleeping difficulties.

Two other studies have examined the psychological adjustment of solvent abusers in non-referred samples. In the study conducted by Nurcombe et al (1970), the Rutter Child Behaviour Questionnaire (Rutter, 1967; Rutter, Tizard and Whitmore, 1970) was completed by teachers at an Aboriginal boys' primary school where petrol sniffing was thought to be common. This study is particularly relevant to the present investigation because the behavioral and emotional problems checklist used here was modeled on the Rutter Child Behavior Questionnaire. The findings were essentially the same as in the present study. Boys who had sniffed petrol were rated as showing greater deviance than their matched, non-sniffing controls on the subscale relating to anti-social conduct (renamed 'tension-discharge' by Nurcombe et al). Scores on the subscale relating to emotional difficulties (renamed 'anxiety-inhibition') were in the same direction but here the difference fell short of statistical significance.

Lavik and Onstad (1986) conducted psychiatric interviews and examined drug use in a sample of 177 adolescents at a junior high school in Norway. The interview focused primarily on emotional difficulties and their data show that marked neurotic symptoms were more common among girls who had tried taking solvents (or other drugs) than among boys who had done so.

Taken together, the results of these two investigations are consistent with those of the present study in suggesting that the types of problems reported by girls who abuse solvents tend to be somewhat different from those reported by boys, with emotional difficulties predominating in the girls and behavioural problems in the boys. This suggestion is consistent with the findings of Skuse and Burrell (1982) who examined cases referred to the Maudsley Hospital Children's Department between 1979 and 1981. Most, but not all, of this group were found to have a psychiatric disorder quite apart from their history of solvent sniffing. The majority of cases had a history of delinquency and many had police records, but emotional disturbance, particularly depression, was also frequently found. Their data show that among the boys, the main diagnoses were conduct disorder in 56% of the cases and emotional disorder in 30%, whereas among the girls 35% were diagnosed as having a conduct disorder and 59% an emotional disorder. The pattern appeared to be the same in both chronic abusers and experimental sniffers.

General population studies of adolescent psychiatric disorders indicate a similar pattern of findings, with emotional disorders occurring more often among girls and conduct disorders occurring more often among boys (Rutter et al, 1976; Rutter, 1979). It therefore seems that the types of psychological problems found among adolescent boys and girls who abuse solvents are similar to those found among adolescents with psychiatric disorders in the general population.

In order to examine whether there was anything distinctive about the types of behavioural and emotional problems shown by adolescents who abuse solvents, they were compared with a sample of controls who had comparably high overall checklist scores. In contrast to the preceding findings, this comparison revealed no marked sex difference in the pattern of problems acknowledged. Solvent abusers of both sexes were more likely to acknowledge conduct problems than controls.

This finding can be taken one step further by asking whether among adolescents with conduct disorders there are any differences in psychological adjustment between those with and without a history of solvent abuse. Most studies that have provided data relevant to this issue have found no differences or have indicated differences only in the degree of disturbance. For example, Biggs, Bender and Foreman (1983) studied boys at a Community Home with Education in London and compared groups matched for age, race and IQ. They found no differences between the two groups on tests of personality, self-concept, locus of control and a projective measure of response to frustration. Dendle (unpublished) studied a sample of girls admitted to a Remand and Assessment Centre in South London in 1981 and compared those who had abused solvents with those who had not. There were only relatively minor differences between the two groups in terms of factors such as history of criminal convictions and number of placements in care, but the solvent abusers were more likely to have made suicidal attempts or gestures and were more
likely to have engaged in minor acts of self-mutilation such as piercing their arms with pins or other sharp objects (an observation also made by Watson (1986)). In addition, they were more likely to have acquired professionally applied tatoos.

Taken together, these findings suggest that although virtually all psychological problems are more common among groups of solvent abusers, what distinguishes their pattern of difficulties from that of other disturbed youngsters is their greater propensity toward delinquent and anti-social problem behaviors. The psychological problems of delinquent solvent abusers do not appear to be markedly different from those of other delinquents, although there is a suggestion that deliberate self-wounding has a more conspicuous profile among the problems of solvent abusers. This last suggestion may be regarded as consistent with the findings of Skuse and Burrell (1982) and Zur and Yule (1990, b) indicating that depression is often an important feature in the psychiatric symptomatology of chronic solvent abusers.

4.4 Neuropsychological Consequences of Solvent Abuse

When the cases and controls were matched for ethnic background as well as school year and sex, there were significant differences between the solvent abusers and their controls on just four of the 35 main test measures. Three of these - the vocabulary subtest, prorated Verbal IQ, and prorated Full Scale IQ - were from the WISC-R. These three scores are not independent of each other: Full Scale IQ is a function of the scores on the tests used to calculate Verbal and Performance IQ, and, in the present study, Verbal IQ was a function of the child's aggregate score on Vocabulary and just one other verbal subtest. The deficit on the verbal subtests could therefore be said to underlie the significant difference observed on Full Scale IQ. The fourth measure which showed a significant difference between groups was from the reaction time task, on which the solvent abusers failed to inhibit an inappropriate response more often than the controls and showed greater variability in response latencies. Taken together the findings suggest that children who abuse solvents tend to have a somewhat lower level of verbal ability and are more impulsive than controls.

In discussing the meaning of these findings, the main question to consider is to what extent these deficits reflect a *causal* effect of solvent abuse. There are several strands of evidence which have a bearing on this issue.

First, the role of adverse social background factors needs to be considered. The domestic circumstances of the solvent abusers were generally less favourable than those of the controls and, as found in numerous other studies, unfavourable domestic circumstances were in turn associated with poor psychological test performance. When multiple regression analyses were carried out to control for the social background differences between groups, none of the four psychological test measures which had previously shown a difference between groups remained statistically significant. A significant difference was found on one other measure - the number of left-right errors on the two-choice reaction time task. However, since this difference had not emerged in the previous uncontrolled comparison between groups, and since it was just one out of a total of 35 significance tests that were carried out, it would be unwise to attach undue significance to this isolated finding.

Second, the *pattern* of test findings needs to be discussed. When groups were matched for ethnic background, the solvent abusers showed a significantly lower mean Verbal IQ than the controls, whereas their Performance IQ deficit was not statistically significant. A similar pattern of test results was obtained by Berry et al (1977), Trites et al (1976) Bigler (1979) and Korman et al (1981) who all found that their solvent abuse groups showed greater impairment in Verbal IQ than in Performance IQ. By contrast, studies of children with a cross-section of neurological disorders (Rutter, Graham and Yule, 1970) or with brain injury due to a variety of particular conditions including hydrocephalus (Dennis, Fitz, Netley et al, 1981), meningitis (Taylor et al, 1984) or head injury (Chadwick et al, 1981 a and b) have consistently shown the opposite pattern of findings, with greater impairment on Performance Scale tasks than in Verbal IQ. Similarly, in studies of detoxified adult alcoholics, impairment has usually been more marked on the subtests of the Performance Scale (Tarter, 1975; Parsons and Farr, 1981; Ron, 1983). Although Verbal-Performance discrepancies of this kind are generally not consistent enough to be useful in the diagnosis of brain injury *in individual cases* (Yule, 1978), the observation of greater impairment on the subtests of Performance scale than on those of the Verbal Scale *in groups* of children with brain injury has been highly consistent. In contrast, the greater deficit on Verbal scale tests, observed in the present study, has been a more typical finding in studies of juvenile delinquents (Wechsler, 1944), poor readers (Rutter, Tizard and Whitmore, 1970) and other groups in which background social disadvantage is a striking feature.

The findings of the present study are in many respects comparable to those from studies of the effects of elevated lead levels on neuropsychological functioning. For example, Smith, Delves, Lansdown, Clayton and Graham (1983) found a

56

statistically significant 5.0 point difference in Full Scale IQ between high and low lead level groups, but this difference ceased to be significant when differences in background social factors were taken into account. Furthermore, most studies of the effects of elevated lead levels have shown greater impairment in Verbal IQ than in Performance IQ (eg, Needleman et al, 1979; Winneke, 1983).

Third, the relationship between the various aspects of the child's sniffing history needs to be considered in relation to the neuropsychological test results. A systematic relationship between the frequency of solvent abuse and performance on the psychological tests - a type of 'dose-response' relationship - would, if present, count as evidence suggestive of a causal effect of solvent abuse on neuropsychological functioning. Similarly, the finding of a relationship between test performance and certain other aspects of the child's sniffing history (eg, the time since the child first started sniffing) might also be taken as evidence for a causal effect. However, the findings from this study provide no clear evidence of any consistent relationship of this kind. After cases and controls who were unmatched for ethnic background had been excluded, there were no significant associations between frequency of solvent abuse and any of the psychological test measures (regardless of how frequency of solvent abuse was categorized). A significant relationship with the other aspects of the child's sniffing history was found only on a few isolated measures (never more than four of the thirty five main measures) and, more often than not, the relationship appeared to be incoherent or inconsistent with the hypothesis of a detrimental effect of solvent abuse.

Fourth, the data relating to changes in test scores over time must be considered. Relative to their test scores prior to solvent abuse, the verbal reasoning quotients of the solvent abusers fell on average by 5.0 points, whereas those of their matched controls increased by 3.3 points. A similarly divergent pattern of change was present in the reading test quotients of the two groups, although, unlike the verbal reasoning test findings, this difference was not statistically significant. At first sight, these longitudinal data apparently indicating deterioration over time, would seem to provide strong evidence that the impaired verbal ability of the solvent abusers was due to solvent abuse.

However, in evaluating the overall significance of these findings, the limitations of the data must be recognised. Antecedent test data for both cases and controls were available for only about half of the case-control pairs and the data that *were* obtained came from a variety of tests, none of which was identical with those used during the course of the study. For example, Verbal IQ, used in the analyses discussed above as a measure equivalent to the antecedent verbal reasoning tests, was a composite measure of scores on the vocabulary and similarities subtests of the WISC-R, and although the similarities subtest might reasonably be considered a measure of verbal reasoning ability, the vocabulary subtest would appear to measure something qualitatively different. In addition, the coherence of the findings is open to question. As is evident from Table 39, the inference that the verbal reasoning test scores of the solvent abusers deteriorated is based on a comparison between one set of findings indicating that their test scores were more than six points *higher* than those of the controls, and another set of findings obtained later showing that their scores were not significantly different from those of the controls. Seen in this light, it is not the deterioration in the performance of the solvent abusers that needs to be explained, but rather their elevated scores prior to solvent abuse. The fact that it is extremely difficult to think of a coherent explanation for the superior test performance of the solvent abusers raises suspicion about the validity of the finding. On the other hand, the pattern of results on the reading test is more comprehensible: the scores of the two groups were similar prior to solvent abuse and diverged subsequently. However, here the decline in scores of the solvent abusers was not statistically significant.

Taken together, the results of the comparisons between test scores obtained before and after solvent abuse are difficult to interpret. In theory, this type of comparison should provide a strong test of the causal hypothesis. The fact that there appeared to be some evidence of deterioration in the performance of the solvent abusers, and the fact that the deterioration was on verbal tests not wholly dissimilar from those on which significant case-control differences were found points to the possibility that the deterioration in scores was real. However, in view of the incomplete nature of the data, the fact that the comparisons are between scores on different types of tests and the indication that the antecedent verbal reasoning test scores produce findings that are in some respects incoherent, the possibility of deterioration cannot be regarded as anything more than a possibility that remains to be convincingly demonstrated.

Putting together these various considerations, it may be concluded that the study provides only very limited support for the idea that solvent abuse causes cognitive impairment and the bulk of the evidence goes against this hypothesis. The solvent abusers showed significant deficits on a few psychological tests, but their impairments were of a type not normally associated with brain damage and could be adequately accounted for in terms of their adverse background domestic circumstances. No relationship was found between psychological test performance and the frequency of solvent abuse and the relationships between test scores and other aspects of the child's sniffing history were generally weak and unsystematic.

It might be objected that this conclusion is merely a reflection of the imperfect sensitivity of the tests used to detect impairment in the present study. This of course is always possible. Only a minority of neuropyschologists would claim that current methods of assessment are optimal and most would point to the need for further investment in research to improve upon existing methods. Nevertheless, it should also be remembered that similar batteries of tests *have* succeeded in demonstrating (a) acute impairment in laboratory studies of samples exposed to comparatively low concentrations of solvents, and (b) persistent deficits in clinical groups such as adult alcoholics (Ron, 1977; Tarter, 1975) or children with various forms of brain damage where a comparable question of impairment has been raised.

Alternatively, it might be objected that the tests used in the present investigation were inappropriate for the detection of those types of impairment which are most likely to result from solvents. Lezak (1986) has recently argued that existing methods of neuropsychological assessment of the effects of industrial toxins have tended to neglect a range of capacities that are difficult to conceptualize, but that broadly fall under the heading of 'executive functions'. These capacities include the capacity to formulate goals, to plan and initiate complex goal-directed activity and to carry out plans effectively and to completion. This point is valid and, as she points out, there is a need to devise methods of assessing functional behaviors of this kind to supplement the tests of cognitive ability currently used. However, Lezak's argument is not that cognitive tests are inappropriate for the detection of effects due to solvents, but rather that they should be supplemented. The cognitive functions that she argues are most likely to be impaired among people exposed to solvents - response speed, memory, attention and concentration - *were* assessed in the present study, but in spite of this no significant impairment attributable to solvent abuse was found.

It might be claimed that the findings underestimate the magnitude of impairment attributable to solvent abuse because pupils who were absent from school on the day the questionnaire was administered were not included in the sample. School absentees include a disproportionate number of drug and solvent abusers (Kandel, 1975; Cooke et al, 1988) and it is likely that frequent solvent abusers are particularly likely to be absent on any given day. However, to some extent, we redressed the resulting underrepresentation of frequent solvent abusers by preferentially selecting for individual assessment pupils who acknowledged frequent solvent abuse. Whilst it is not possible to say whether the frequency of solvent abuse in our selected cases precisely reflects the frequency of the practice in the combined population of school attenders and absentees, we believe that it was probably not markedly different. In spite of the strong association between school absenteeism and drug abuse, only a minority of absentees abuse drugs and probably only a minority of this minority are frequent drug users.

Nevertheless, it is important to emphasize the limits to the generalizability of the present findings. The pattern of solvent abuse among the cases we studied could best be described as predominantly experimental or occasional, with only a minority reporting a history of frequent or habitual abuse. Our findings cannot necessarily be generalized to samples whose experience of the practice is more frequent or prolonged or to cases who have abused different products. Similarly, it would be wrong to infer from our findings that occasional solvent abuse is a harmless practice. It is not. At least 10% of 13 to 16 year old solvent abuse deaths involve youngsters abusing for the first time (Anderson, Bloor and Ramsey, unpublished data). Nevertheless, the finding that solvent abuse, as commonly practiced by secondary school pupils, is unlikely to result in neuropsychological impairment is reassuring. As such, it should contribute to the informed clinical assessment of adolescents who present with a history of occasional solvent abuse as well as to the counseling of those youngsters and parents who are unduly worried about he damage that might have been done.

5 Summary of Main Findings

In a representative sample of over 4000 third, fourth and fifth year secondary school pupils, 3.6% acknowledged having abused solvents to the point of intoxication. This proportion is almost certainly an underestimate of the true prevalence of solvent abuse because it does not take into account false negative questionnaire responses, and it neglects the higher rate of solvent abuse among school absentees.

Although studies of fatalities and clinic referrals associated with solvent abuse have generally reported a marked excess of boys, in the present study there was no sex difference in the prevalence of solvent abuse among children attending co-educational schools. Several possible reasons were put forward to explain the male preponderance among fatalities and clinic referrals. Consistent with the findings of other studies, a peak in the prevalence of solvent abuse was noted among fourth year pupils (aged 14 to 15 years).

As in other population-based surveys, in the majority of those who sniffed the pattern of solvent abuse could best be described as experimental. Nearly half of those who had abused solvents had done so only once or twice and nearly four-fifths had sniffed fewer than ten times. Only about one in thirteen had sniffed more than 30 times.

Typewriter correction fluids were the most popularly abused products in the present investigation and had been tried by approximately two-thirds of the solvent abusers. Various glues and butane gas had each been abused by roughly a third of the cases. Other substances such as dry-cleaning fluids, petrol, amyl nitrite, paints and aerosols had also been tried by a few children, but in each case by less than 5% of the cases. Nearly half of the solvent abusers had sniffed more than one product and just over 10% had tried three or more different products.

Solvents were detected in the breath of one in fifteen of the cases who acknowledged solvent abuse (ever) and, for reasons that are unclear, in one of the 106 controls. In all cases, the substance identified was consistent with the product reported to have been abused most recently.

Half of the solvent abusers in the present investigation could be described as current sniffers in as much as they had abused solvents during the six months prior to the initial assessment. However, generally speaking, the practice was of recent onset and was unlikely to persist. In approximately half of the cases, solvents had first been abused during the 12 months before the study was conducted, and fewer than one in five had first sniffed more than 2 years beforehand. More than three-quarters of those who were traced and examined at follow-up had not abused solvents during the 9 month interval between the two assessments.

There were marked difference between the solvent abusers and the control group in levels of cigarette smoking and drinking and in their use of illicit drugs. Not only were all classes of drugs more likely to have been used by the solvents abusers, but they were more likely to have been used frequently and recently. The differences with respect to cigarette and cannabis smoking were particularly marked.

The background domestic circumstances of the solvent abusers were generally less favorable than those of the general population controls, but these differences were not nearly as marked as those found in studies of clinical referrals. The solvent abusers were significantly more likely than the controls to be members of large sibships and to come from homes in which neither parent was employed. In addition, there were significantly fewer black children and more white children in the sample of solvent abusers than among the randomly selected controls.

Although the study produced little evidence that school children who abuse solvents suffer from more physical illnesses than others, they were more likely to complain of coughing and shortness of breath. Lung function tests, however, showed no significant differences between groups. The solvent abusers were more likely to sustain accidental injuries requiring hospital treatment between the initial and follow-up assessments.

The solvent abusers were significantly more likely to acknowledge current behavioral and emotional problems than the controls. The types of problems acknowledged appeared to be similar to those found in general population studies of adolescents with psychiatric disorders, with conduct problems occurring more often among the boys and emotional problems among the girls. However, when the solvent abusers were compared with controls who had comparably high levels of self-reported psychological problems, it appeared that what was distinctive about the pattern of problems of the solvent abusers (both male and female) was their greater propensity toward delinquent and anti-social behaviors.

The evidence from this study suggests that solvent abuse, as commonly practiced by secondary school pupils, is unlikely to cause neuropsychological impairment. When cases and controls were matched for ethnic background, the solvent abusers were found to have a mean Full Scale IQ that was 5.4 points below that of the controls, a statistically significant difference. Their performance on tests of vocabulary, Verbal IQ and a measure of impulsivity also showed significant impairment. However, when differences between groups in social background circumstances were partialled out statistically, none of these four measures continued to show a significant effect. Evidence for deterioration over time was unconvincing. In addition, there was no significant effect of frequency of solvent abuse on any of the outcome measures, and the effects of factors such as recency of solvent abuse, type and number of products abused and time since solvents had first been abused were generally either non-significant or unsystematic.

Appendix A

Self-completed Screening Questionnaire

CONFIDENTIAL

ST GEORGE'S HOSPITAL MEDICAL SCHOOL

SCHOOLS HEALTH SURVEY

 We are carrying out a survey at a number of schools because we
are interested in various things that may affect the health and
educational progress of young people.
We would be grateful if you would help us by completing this
questionnaire.

PLEASE ANSWER ALL OF THE QUESTIONS

ALL OF YOUR ANSWERS WILL BE **CONFIDENTIAL** AND
YOUR PARENTS AND TEACHERS WILL **NOT** SEE OR BE
TOLD ABOUT YOUR ANSWERS TO ANY OF THE QUESTIONS.

PLEASE WRITE IN BLOCK CAPITALS

YOUR DATE OF BIRTH...

YOUR TUTOR GROUP...

PLEASE WRITE IN BLOCK CAPITALS

YOUR FIRST NAME(S): ....

YOUR LAST NAME: ....

---

1. How old are you? ....

2. Are you a boy or a girl? *Tick one*

   i) Boy ☐

   ii) Girl ☐

3. With whom do you live most of the time? *Tick one*

   i) Both parents ☐

   ii) Father only ☐

   iii) Mother only ☐

   iv) Father and stepmother ☐

   v) Mother and stepfather ☐

   vi) Foster parents ☐

   vii) Other relatives ☐

   viii) Others (not relatives) ☐

4. Altogether how many people usually live at home, including yourself? ....

5. Do you and your family live in a house or a flat?

Tick one

   i) House

   ii) Flat/Maisonette

   iii) Other

6. Does your family own your home or is it rented?

Tick one

   i) Owned or paying a mortgage

   ii) Rented from council

   iii) Rented, but not from council

   iv) Other (eg rent free)

7. How many bedrooms are there in your home? ....

8. What type of heating do you use at home?

Tick all that apply

   i) None

   ii) Paraffin

   iii) Gas fire

   iv) Electric

   v) Central heating

   vi) Other

   (Please say...)

9. Have you **ever** missed school for **more than a month** at a time because of illness or accident?

Tick one

   i) Yes

   ii) No

10. **During the past month,** how many school days have you missed because of illness?

Tick one

   i) None ☐

   ii) One ☐

   iii) Two or three ☐

   iv) Four or more ☐

11. Do you **usually** cough first thing in the morning?

Tick one

   i) Yes ☐

   ii) No ☐

12. Do you **usually** cough during the day or at night?

Tick one

   i) Yes ☐

   ii) No ☐

13. Do you get short of breath when hurrying on level ground or walking up a slight hill?

Tick one

   i) Yes ☐

   ii) No ☐

14. **During the last 12 months,** have you suffered from any of the following?

Tick all that apply

   i) Asthma or wheeziness in the chest ☐

   ii) Bronchitis or pneumonia ☐

   iii) Hayfever ☐

   iv) Eczema ☐

We also want to ask about a few things that may affect your health.

15. Have you ever smoked a cigarette?

Tick one

   i) Yes ☐

   ii) No ☐

---

16. When did you last have a cigarette?

Tick one

   i) Earlier today ☐

   ii) Yesterday ☐

   iii) Two or three days ago ☐

   iv) More than three days ago, but during the past week ☐

   v) More than a week ago, but during the past month ☐

   vi) More than a month ago, but during the last 12 months ☐

   vii) More than a year ago ☐

   viii) Never ☐

---

17. How often do you smoke now?

Tick one

   i) Not at all ☐

   ii) One or two cigarettes occasionally ☐

   iii) Several cigarettes a week, but not every day ☐

   iv) One or two cigarettes a day ☐

   v) More than two cigarettes, but not more than 10 a day ☐

   vi) More than 10 cigarettes a day, but not more than 20 a day ☐

   vii) More than 20 cigarettes a day ☐

---

18. If you smoke now, please write down the names of all the brands of cigarettes that you smoke regularly.

....

....

19. When you have a cigarette, do you inhale and take the smoke right down into your lungs?

Tick one

   i) Yes ☐

   ii) No ☐

   iii) I do not smoke ☐

---

20. Does your father (or stepfather) smoke at home?

Tick one

   i) Yes ☐

   ii) No ☐

   iii) No father or stepfather at home ☐

---

21. Does your mother (or stepmother) smoke at home?

Tick one

   i) Yes ☐

   ii) No ☐

   iii) No mother or stepmother at home ☐

---

22. Have you ever sniffed glue, solvents or anything else on purpose?

Tick one

   i) Yes ☐

   ii) No ☐

If "yes"

a) Please write down the names of everything you have ever sniffed or inhaled.

....

....

b) Have you ever sniffed enough to feel "high" or intoxicated?

Tick one

   i) Yes ☐

   ii) No ☐

   iii) Don't know ☐

23. How often have you sniffed glue (or anything else) on purpose?

Tick one

   i) Not at all ☐

   ii) Once or twice ☐

   iii) Three or four times ☐

   iv) About 5 - 9 times ☐

   v) About 10 - 30 times ☐

   vi) More than 30 times ☐

24. When did you last sniff glue (or anything else) on purpose?

Tick one

   i) Earlier today ☐

   ii) Yesterday ☐

   iii) Two or three days ago ☐

   iv) More than three days ago, but during the past week ☐

   v) More than a week ago, but during the past month ☐

   vi) More than a month ago, but during the past year ☐

   vii) More than a year ago ☐

   viii) Never ☐

25. Have you ever drunk any alcohol?

Tick one

   i) Yes ☐

   ii) No ☐

If "yes"

Have you ever had enough alcohol to feel drunk?

Tick one

   i) No ☐

   ii) Not "drunk", but enough to feel slightly tipsy ☐

   iii) Yes ☐

26. When did you last have an alcoholic drink?   *Tick one*

   i) Earlier today ☐

   ii) Yesterday ☐

   iii) Two or three days ago ☐

   iv) More than three days ago, but during the last week ☐

   v) More than a week ago, but during the last month ☐

   vi) More than a month ago, but during the last 12 months ☐

   vii) More than a year ago ☐

   viii) Never ☐

27. During the last 12 months, approximately how often have you
had an alcoholic drink?   *Tick one*

   i) Never ☐

   ii) Christmas & special occasions only ☐

   iii) Less than once a month ☐

   iv) At least once a month, but less than once a week ☐

   v) Once or twice a week ☐

   vi) More than once or twice a week, but not every day ☐

   vii) Every day ☐

28. Please write down the name of anything alcoholic you have had in
the last month.

....

....

29. **During the last 12 months,** have you:

	Never	Rarely	Sometimes	Often
i) Had trouble falling asleep or staying asleep?	☐	☐	☐	☐
ii) Missed meals because you just didn't feel like eating anything?	☐	☐	☐	☐
iii) Suffered from stomach aches?	☐	☐	☐	☐
iv) Suffered from headaches?	☐	☐	☐	☐
v) Felt very tense or nervous?	☐	☐	☐	☐
vi) Had difficulties concentrating on school work?	☐	☐	☐	☐
vii) Worried a lot	☐	☐	☐	☐
viii) Been teased or bullied at school?	☐	☐	☐	☐
ix) Been involved in fights with other boys or girls?	☐	☐	☐	☐
x) Stolen something that didn't belong to you?	☐	☐	☐	☐
xi) Deliberately damaged something that didn't belong to you?	☐	☐	☐	☐
xii) Stayed away from school or left school early when you should have been there?	☐	☐	☐	☐
xiii) Felt very miserable or unhappy?	☐	☐	☐	☐
xiv) Felt very lonely?	☐	☐	☐	☐
xv) Been worried about your health?	☐	☐	☐	☐

(If you have been worried about your health, please explain) ....

....

....

....

....

30. How do you travel to school?

Tick all that apply

   i) Walk ☐

  ii) Bicycle ☐

 iii) Bus ☐

 iv) Train (main line) ☐

  v) Tube ☐

 vi) Car ☐

31. Outside school hours how much time do you spend on sports or physical activities such as cycling, running, swimming etc?

Tick one

   i) None or less than an hour a week ☐

  ii) About 1 or 2 hours week ☐

 iii) About 3 - 5 hours a week ☐

 iv) About 6 - 10 hours a week ☐

  v) More than 10 hours a week ☐

Thank you for your help in answering these questions.

If you wish to make any other comments about your health or anything else, please write below.

Appendix B

Psychological Test Battery
(Initial Assessment)

Wechsler Intelligence Scale for Children - Revised (WISC-R)
(Wechsler, 1974)
An abbreviated version of the WISC-R was used to provide a measure of intellectual ability. Four subtests were used: two from the Verbal Scale (Similarities and Vocabulary) and two from the Performance Scale (Picture Completion and Block Design). These subtests were selected from the ten that comprise the full test because of a) their high correlations with Full Scale IQ, b) their satisfactory reliability and stability over time, and c) their brevity (Kaufman, 1979).

EH-3 Reading Test (NFER)
The EH-3 provides a measure of reading comprehension speed. The task involves silent reading of two prose passages in which some words have been replaced by five different 'answer' words. Comprehension is assessed by requiring the subject to underline the one that fits best with the sense of the passage. The raw score is obtained by counting the number of multiple choice items completed in the time available for reading (4.5 min). A reading quotient can be derived from tables of age-specific normative data.

Passage Recall
A fifty- four word news story reporting an oil tanker accident (Applied Psychology Unit, Cambridge, Unpublished) was read to the subject. Recall was tested immediately afterwards and again after an interval of 45 minutes, during which time the tests listed below were administered.

Speed of Information Processing - Version E
(British Ability Scales, 1983)
The subject is presented with a 5 x 5 item array of numbers and is required to indicate the highest number on each row as quickly as possible. The test comprises ten such arrays. The task difficulty increases over the course of the test as the numbers become longer and the differences between them more difficult to distinguish. Age-specific normative data are published to permit conversion of the raw score to a T-score (with a mean of 50 and a standard deviation of 7).

Bexley-Maudsley Automated Screening Tests (BMAPS)
(Acker and Acker, 1982)
BMAPS was developed for neuropsychological assessment of chronic alcoholics. It comprises five separate subtests. The tests have been shown to discriminate between groups of detoxified adult alcoholics and controls (Acker and Acker,

1982) and Zur and Yule (in press, a) found significant differences between chronic solvent abusers and delinquents on two of the subtests. These two were used in the present study.

(a)   **Visual Perceptual Analysis**
        Three geometrical patterns, each consisting of 20 elements, are presented on the computer monitor. The subject is required to indicate which pattern is different from the other two as quickly as possible. Feedback (correct/wrong) is presented automatically after each of 24 trials. On 12 trials, the patterns differ in four of the 20 elements (easy items);   on the other 12 randomly interspersed trials they differ only on two of them (difficult items). The test was designed to measure perceptuo-motor speed.

 (b)   **Symbol-Digit Coding Test**
        This is a computerised adaptation of the Digit Symbol Coding subtest of the WISC-R. A visual key, linking the numbers 1 to 9 with nine different geometrical symbols, is present on the screen throughout the duration of the task. Immediately above, the symbols are presented one at a time in random order. The subject is required to respond by pressing the key of the corresponding number as quickly as possible. The version used in the initial assessment consisted of forty-five items.

Automated Psychological Test System (Elithorn and Levander, unpublished)
  (a) **Reaction Time Tests**
        Reaction time (RT) tests have been found to be sensitive to a variety of types of brain damage (eg, Blackburn and Benton, 1955; Miller, 1970) as well as to exposure to various solvents (Gamberale, 1976). Three forms of reaction time (RT) task were used: (i) simple unprepared visual RT; (ii) two-choice visual RT; (iii) two-choice visual RT 'with inhibition'. This last form of the test is similar to (ii), except that the subject is required to *withhold* a response on trials when a tone is presented at the same time as the visual stimulus. It was included because of evidence that some children with brain damage may have difficulty withholding inappropriate responses (Brown, Chadwick, Shaffer, Rutter and Traub 1981).

 (b)   **Finger Tapping Tasks**
        A special four-key response console was used to measure   the subject's speed of finder tapping during an 8 second period using: (i) Right index finger; (ii)left index finger; (iii) right index and middle fingers alternating; (iv) left index and middle fingers alternating; (v) right and left index fingers alternating.

 (c)   **Trial-Making Tasks**
        An automated version of Armitage's (1946) test in which the subject had to use a joystick on the response console in order to move the cursor to 'hit'

each target in turn. Two forms of the task were used. The targets were (i) The numbers 1 to 9 in order; (ii) The letters A to I and the numbers 1 to 9 in alternating sequence (ie, A, 1, B, 2, C . . . . .9).

Manual Dexterity Task (Annett, 1970)
The subject is required to move ten doweling pegs from one row to holes to another as quickly as possible. Five trails are allowed with each hand. The test involves both gross visuo-motor coordination and fine motor skills.

Vibration Perception Threshold
Some industrial workers exposed to solvents have been found to show a form of sensory imperception involving impairment of touch and vibration perception (Elofsson et al, 1980; Husman and Karli, 1980). The same has been found in a few chronic solvent abusers (Malm and Lying-Tunnell, 1980). Vibration perception thresholds were measured in the present study using a portable Biothesiometer (BioMedical Instrument Co, Newbury, Ohio) - a hand-held mains-operated device with a 100 Hz vibrating rubber tactor- which was applied at right angles to the palmar aspect of the thumb opposite the nail-bed and medial malleolus of the subject's non-preferred limb. The amplitude of vibration was gradually increased from zero until the subject reported detection of the sensation. The threshold of perception was taken as the median of three trials at each site.

Appendix C

Psychological Tests Introduced for Follow-up Assessment

British Picture Vocabulary Scale
(Dunn, Dunn, Whetton & Pintilie, 1982)

The subject is required to indicate which of a set of four line drawings best illustrates the meaning of a stimulus word which is spoken by the examiner. The short (38 item) version of the test was used in the present study. It provides a measure of vocabulary which is relatively independent of the subject's ability to express himself in words.

Matching Familiar Figures Test
(Kagan, Rosman, Day, Albert & Phillips, 1964)

The subject is required to select from a set of six very similar line drawings the one that is identical to a simultaneously presented stimulus figure. Ten sets of figures are presented and the response time and the number of errors on each of them are recorded. Short latency incorrect responses are interpreted as a reflection of an 'impulsive' cognitive style.

Spiral Maze Test (Gibson, 1977)

The subject is required to draw his way out of a spiral-shaped maze as quickly as possible. There are a number of 'obstacles' along the path and he is warned about not crossing either these or the edges of the path with his pencil. Time-stress is created by sharply reminding the subject every 15 seconds to go as quickly as possible. The total time taken to trace the maze and the number of errors are recorded. Delinquents have been found to perform this test more quickly and more carelessly than others.

References

Abelson HI, Fishburne PM, Cisin I.
National Survey on Drug Abuse:: DHEW Publ No (ADM) 78-618, US Government Printing Office, Washington DC 1977

Acker W, Acker C.
The Bexley-Maudsley Automated Screening Test.
NFER-Nelson Publishing Co: Windsor, Berkshire, 1982

Ackerley WC, Gibson G.
Lighter fluid sniffing.
Amer J Psychiat 1964; 120: 1056-1061

Allison WM, Jerrom DWA.
Glue sniffing: a pilot study of the cognitive effects of long-term use.
Int J Addict 1984; 19: 453-458

Altenkirch H, Mager J, Stoltenburg G, Helmbrecht J.
Toxic polyneuropathies after sniffing a glue thinner.
J Neurol 1977; 214: 137-152

American Thoracic Society: ATS Statement.
Snowbird workshop on standardization of spirometry.
Amer Rev Resp Dis 1979; 119: 831-838

Anderson HR, Macnair RS, Ramsey JD.
Deaths from abuse of volatile substances: A national epidemiological study.
Brit Med J 1985; 290: 304-307

Annett M.
The growth of manual preference and speed.
Brit J Psychol 1970; 61: 545-558

Armitage SG.
An analysis of certain psychological tests used for the evaluation of brain injury.
Psychol Monog 1946; 60: Whole No 277

Axelson O, Hane M, Hogstedt C.
A case-referent study of neuropsychiatric disorders among workers exposed to solvents.
Scand J Work Environ Health 1976; 2: 14-20

Baker EL, Fine LJ.
Solvent neurotoxicity: the current evidence.
J Occup Med 1986; 28: 126-129

Barker G, Adams W.
Glue sniffing.
Sociol Soc Res 1963; 47: 289-310

Bass M.
Sudden sniffing death.
JAMA 1970; 212: 2075-2079

Bate SM.
Reading Test EH-3.
National Foundation for Educational Research:
Windsor, Berkshire, 1970.

Beauvais F, Oetting ER, Edwards RW.
Trends in drug use of Indian adolescents living
on reservations: 1975-1983.
Amer J Drug Alcohol Abuse 1985; 11: 209-229 (a)

Beauvais F, Oetting ER, Edwards RW.
Trends in the use of inhalants among American Indian adolescents.
White Cloud Journal 1985; 3: 3-11 (b)

Berry GJ.
Neuropsychological assessment of chronic solvent abusers: A preliminary report
to the National Institute on Drug Abuse. Washington, DC: US Government
Printing Office, 1976.

Berry GJ, Heaton RK, Kirby MW.
Neuropsychological deficits of chronic inhalant abusers.
In Rumack BM, Temple AR (Eds) Management of the poisoned patient.
Princeton, N J, 1977

Bethell MF.
Toxic psychosis caused by inhalation of petrol fumes.
Brit Med J 1965; ii, 276-277

Biggs SJ, Bender MP, Foreman J.
Are there psychological differences between persistent solvent-abusing delin-
quents and delinquents who do not abuse solvents?
J Adolesc 1983; 6: 71-86

Bigler ED.
Neuropsychological evaluation of adolescent patients hospitalised with chronic inhalant abuse.
Clin Neuropsychol 1979; 1: 8-12

Blackburn HL, Benton AL.
Simple and choice reaction time in cerebral disease.
Confinia Neurol 1955; 15: 327-338

Boeckx RL, Postl B, Coodin FS.
Gasoline sniffing and tetra-ethyl lead poisoning in children.
Pediat 1977, 60: 140-145

Boor JW, Hurtig HJ.
Persistent cerebellar ataxia after exposure to toluene.
Ann Neurol 1977; 2: 440-442

Brecher E.
Licit and illicit drugs.
Little, Brown and Co, Boston and Toronto 1974

Brown G, Chadwick O, Shaffer D, Rutter M, Traub M.
A prospective study of children with head injuries:
III Psychiatric sequelae.
Psychol Med 1981; 11: 63-78

Brozovsky M, Winkler EG.
Glue sniffing in children and adolescents.
NY J Med 1965; 65: 1984-1989

Castro ME, Valencia M.
Drug consumption among the student population of Mexico City and its metropolitan area: subgroups affected and the distribution of users.
Bull Narcotics 1980; 32: 29-37

Chadwick O, Rutter M.
Neuropsychological assessment.
In Rutter M, (Ed): Developmental Neuropsychiatry.
Guilford: New York, 1983

Chadwick O, Rutter M, Brown G, Shaffer D, Traub M.
A prospective study of children with head injuries:
II Cognitive sequelae.
Psychol Med 1981; 11: 49-61 (a)

Chadwick O, Rutter M, Shaffer D, Shrout PE.
A prospective study of children with head injuries:
IV Specific cognitive deficits.
J Clin Neuropsychol 1981; 3: 101-120 (b)

Cherry N, Hutchins H, Pace T, Waldron HA.
Neurobehavioural effects of repeated occupational exposure to toluene and paint solvents.
Brit J Ind Med 1985; 42: 291-300

Clark DG, Tinston DJ.
Acute inhalation toxicity of halogenated and non-halogenated hydrocarbons.
Hum Toxicol 1982; 1: 239-247

Clinger OW, Johnson NA.
Purposeful inhalation of gasoline fumes.
Psychiat Quart 1951; 25: 357

Cohen S.
The volatile solvents.
Pub Health Rev 1973; 11: 185-214

Cohen S.
Inhalants and solvents.
In: Youth Drug Abuse : Problems, Issues and Treatment. Beschner GM
and Friedman AS (Eds): Lexington, MA: D C Heath, 1979.

Cooke BRB, Evans DA, Farrow SC.
Solvent misuse in secondary school children - a prevelence study.
Comm Med 1988; 10: 8-13.

Dendle J.
Glue-sniffing and solvent abuse among adolescent girls.
Report of research carried out at Cumberlow Lodge Remand and Assessment Centre for Girls' during 1980 and 1981.
London Borough of Lambeth, unpublished.

Dennis M, Fitz CR, Netley CT, Sugar J, Harwood-Nash DCF, Hendrick EB, Hoffman HJ, Humphreys RP.
The intelligence of hydrocephalic children.
Arch Neurol 1981; 38: 607-615

Diamond ID, Pritchard C, Choudry N, Fielding M, Cox M, Bushnell D.
The incidence of drug and solvent misuse among Southern English normal comprehensive school children.
Pub Health 1988; 102: 107-114.

Dodds J, Santostefano S.
A comparison of the cognitive functioning of glue-sniffers and non-sniffers.
J Pediat 1964; 64: 565-570

Dunn L, Dunn L, Whetton C, Pintile D.
British Picture Vocabulary Scale.
NFER-Nelson: Windsor, 1982

Dunoon D, Homel P.
Solvent and aerosol abuse in New South Wales.
Report AB4/1: New South Wales Drug and Alcohol Authority Sydney, 1984

Ehyai A, Freemon FR.
Progressive optic neuropathy and sensori-neural hearing loss due to chronic glue
sniffing.
J Neurol Neurosurg Psychiat 1983; 46: 349-351

Elithorn A, Levander S.
Automated Psychological Test System
Unpublished

Elliot C, Murray DJ, Pearson LS.
The British Ability Scales.
National Foundation for Educational Research: Windsor, Berkshire 1983.

Elofsson GA, Gamberale F, Hindmarsh T, Iregren A,
Isaksson A, Johnsson I, Knave B, Lydahl E, Mindus P, Persson HE, Philipson B,
Steby M, Struwe G, Soderman E, Wennberg A, Widen L.
Exposure to organic solvents.
Scand J Work Environ Health 1980; 6: 239-273

Faber P.
No passing fashion: The East Sussex solvent abuse study.
Unpublished, 1985

Faucett RL, Jensen RA.
Addiction to the inhalation of gasoline fumes in a child.
J Pediat 1952; 41: 364

Fejer D, Smart RG, Whitehead PC.
Changes in the patterns of drug use in two Canadian cities: Toronto and Halifax
Int J Addict 1972; 7: 467-479

Filskov SB, Golstein SG.
Diagnostic validity of the Halstead-Reitan Neuropsychological Battery.
J Consult Clin Psychol 1974; 42: 382-388

Finlayson MAJ, Johnson KA, Reitan RM.
Relationship of level of education to neuropsychological measures in brain-damaged and non-brain-damaged adults.
J Consult Clin Psychol 1977; 45: 536-542

Fishburne PM, Abelson HI, Cisin I.
National survey on drug abuse: Main findings 1979.
Rockville, MD, National Institute on Drug Abuse, 1980
DHHS Publ (ADM) 80-976: US Government

Fornazzari L, Wilkinson DA, Kapur BM, Carlen PL.
Cerebellar, cortical and functional impairment in toluene abusers.
Acta Neurol Scand 1983; 67: 319-329

Gamberale F.
Behavioural effects of exposure to solvent vapors: experimental and field studies.
In Horvath M (Ed) Adverse effects of environmental chemicals and psychotropic Drugs. Elsevier: Amsterdam, 1976

Gibson HB.
Manual of the Spiral Maze Test, 2nd Ed.
Hodder and Stoughton Educational: Sevenoaks, 1977

Glaser HH, Massengale ON.
Glue-sniffing in children.
JAMA 1962; 181: 300-303

Golden CJ, Moses JA, Fishburne FJ, Engum E, Lewis GP, Wisniewski AM, Conley FK, Berg RA, Graber B.
Cross-validation of the Luria-Nebraska Neuropsychological Battery for the presence, lateralization and localization of brain damage.
J Consult Clin Psychol 1981; 49: 491-507

Gossett JT, Lewis JM, Phillips VA.
Extent and prevalence of illicit drug use as reported by 56,745 students.
JAMA 1971; 216: 1464-1470

Grabski DA.
Toluene sniffing producing cerebellar degeneration.
Amer J Psychiat 1961; 118: 461-462

Hall DMB, Ramsey J, Schwarz MS, Dookun D.
Neuropathy in a petrol sniffer.
Arch Dis Child 1986; 61: 900-901

Halstead WC.
Brain and Intelligence.
University of Chicago Press: Chicago, 1947

Herbert M.
The concept and testing of brain damage in children:
A review.
J Child Psychol Psychiat 1964; 5: 197-216

Husman K, Karli P.
Clinical neurological findings among car painters exposed to a mixture of organic
solvents.
Scand J Work Environ Health 1980; 6: 33-39

Institute for the Study of Drug Dependence.
Survey and Statistics on Drugtaking in Britain.
ISDD Library and Information Service, London 1986

Jessor R, Jessor SL.
Problem Behavior and Psychosocial Development.
Academic Press: New York 1977

Johnson KG, Donnelly JH, Scheble R, Wine RL, Weitman M.
Survey of adolescent drug use: I Sex and grade distribution.
Am J Public Health 1971; 61: 2418-2434

Johnston LD, O'Malley PM, Bachman JG.
Drugs and American High School Students 1975-1983.
Rockville, MD, National Institute on Drug Abuse, 1984
US Department of Health and Human Services

Kagan J, Rosman BL, Day D, Albert J, Phillips W.
Information processing in the child: Significance of analytic and reflective
attitudes.
Psychol Monog 1964; 78: 1-37

Kandel D.
Reaching the hard-to-reach: Illicit drug use among high school absentees.
Addict Dis 1975; 1: 465-480

Kandel D, Single E, Kessler RC.
The epidemiology of drug use among New York State High School Students:
Distribution, trends and changes in rates of use.
Amer J Pub Health 1976; 66: 43-53

Kaufman A.
Gasoline sniffing among children in a Pueblo Indian village. Paediat 1973; 51:
1060-1064

Kaufman AS.
Intelligent testing with the WISC-R.
Wiley-Interscience: New York, 1979

King MD, Day RE, Oliver JS, Lush M, Watson JM.
Solvent encephalopathy.
Brit Med J 1981; 283: 663-665

Korman M, Matthews RW, Lovitt R.
Neuropsychological effects of abuse of inhalants.
Percept Mot Skills 1981; 53: 547-553

Korobkin R, Ashbury AK, Sumner AJ, Neilsen SL.
Glue-sniffing neuropathy.
Arch Neurol 1975; 32: 158-162

Knave B, Anselm Olson B, Elofsson A, Gamberale F,
Isaksson A, Mindus P, Persson HE, Struwe G, Wennberg A, Westerholm P.
Long-term exposure to jet fuel: A cross-sectional epidemiologic investigation on
occupationally exposed industrial workers with special reference to the nervous
system.
Scand J Work Environ Health 1978; 4: 19-45

Knox JW, Nelson JR.
Permanent encephalopathy from toluene.
N Eng J Med 1966; 275: 1494-1496

Lavik NJ, Onstad S.
Drug use and psychiatric symptoms in adolescence.
Acta Psychiat Scand 1986; 73: 437-440

Lawton JJ, Malmquist CP.
Gasoline addiction in children.
Psychiat Quart 1961; 35: 555-561

Lezak MD.
Neuropsychological assessment in behavioural toxicology - developing techniques and interpretive issues.
Scand J Work Environ Health 1984; 10: Suppl. 1, 25-29.

Lindstrom K, Riihimaki H, Hanninen K.
Occupational solvent exposure and neuropyschiatric disorders.
Scand J Work Environ Health 1984; 10: 321-3

London Reading Test: Teacher's Manual.
ILEA and NFER-Nelson: Windsor, 1980

Lynch P.
Interim report on the findings of the survey into solvent misuse by schoolchildren in Berkshire.
Unpublished, 1984

Mahmood Z.
Cognitive functioning of solvent abusers.
Scot Med J, 1983; 28: 276-280

Malm G, Lying-Tunnell U.
Cerebellar dysfunction related to toluene sniffing.
Acta Neurol Scand 1980; 62: 188-190

Massengale ON, Glaser HH, LeLievre RE, Dodds JB, Klock ME.
Physical and psychologic factors in glue-sniffing.
N Eng J Med 1963; 29: 1340-1344

May PA.
Substance abuse and American Indians: Prevalence and susceptibility.
Int J Addict 1982; 17: 1185-1209

Merrill E.
Sniffing solvents.
Pepar Publications: Birmingham, 1985

Merry J, Zachariadis N.
Addiction to glue sniffing.
Brit Med J 1962; ii: 1448

Mikkelsen S.
A cohort study of disability pension and death among painters with special regard to disabling pre-senile dementia as occupational disease.
Scand J Soc Med 1980; 16: 34-43

Miller E.
Simple and choice reaction time following severe head injury.
Cortex 1970; 6: 121-127

Ministry of Education
Report on the Survey of Drug Use among Victorian Postprimary Students.
Ministry of Education, Victoria, Australia, 1986

Nagle DR.
Anaesthetic addiction and drunkenness: a contemporary and historical survey.
Int J Addict 1968; 3: 25-39

Needleman H, Gunnoe C, Leviton A, Reed R, Peresie H,
Maher C, Barrett BS.
Deficits in psychologic and classroom performance of children with elevated
dentine lead levels.
N Eng J Med 1979; 300: 689-695

National Opinion Polls Market research Ltd.
Survey of drug abuse in the 15-21 age group undertaken for the Daily Mail.
NOP: London, 1982

Novak A.
The deliberate inhalation of volatile substances.
J Psychedelic Drugs 1980; 12: 105-122

Nurcombe B, Bianchi G, Money J, Cawte J.
A hunger for stimuli: The psychosocial background of petrol inhalation.
Brit J Med Psychol, 1970; 43: 367-374

Nylander I.
"Thinner" addiction in children and adolescents.
Acta Paedopsychiat 1962; 29: 273-283

Oetting ER, Edwards R, Goldstein GS, Garcia-Mason V.
Drug use among adolescents of five southwestern native
American tribes.
Int J Addict 1980; 15: 439-445

Oldham W.
Deliberate self-intoxication with petrol vapour.
Brit Med J 1961; 2: 1687-1688

Olsen J, Sabroe S.
A case-referent study of neuropsychiatric disorders among workers exposed to solvents in the Danish wood and furniture industry.
Scand J Soc Med 1980; 16: 44-49

Parker MJ, Tarlow MJ and Anderson JM.
Glue sniffing and cerebral infarction.
Arch Dis Child 1984; 59: 675-677

Parsons OA, Farr SP.
The neuropsychology of alcohol and drug use.
In Filskov SB, Boll TJ (Eds) Handbook of Clinical Neuropsychology.
Wiley: New York, 1981

Perez R, Padilla AM, Ramirez A, Ramirez R, Rodriguez M.
Correlation and changes over time in drug and alcohol use within a barrio population.
Amer J Comm Psychol 1980; 8: 621-636

Plant MA, Peck DF, Stuart R.
The correlates of serious alcohol-related consequence and illicit drug use amongst a cohort of Scottish teenagers.
Brit J Addict 1984; 79: 197-200

Plant MA, Peck DF, Samuel E.
Alcohol, Drugs and School-leavers.
Tavistock: London, 1985

Porter MR, Vieira TA, Kaplan GJ, Heesch JR, Colyar AB.
Drug use in Anchorage, Alaska: A survey of 15,634 students in grades 6 through 12 - 1971.
JAMA 1973; 223: 657-664

Preble E, Laury GV.
Plastic cement: The ten cent hallucinogen.
Int J Addictions 1967; 2: 271-281

Press E, Done AK.
Solvent sniffing: Physiological effects and community control measures for intoxication from the intentional inhalation of organic solvents.
I Pediat 1967; 39: 451-461
II Pediat 1967; 39: 611-622

Prigitano GP, Parsons OA.
Relationship of age and education to Halstead Test performance in different patient populations.
J Consult Clin Psychol 1976; 44: 527-533

Pritchard C, Fielding M, Choudry N, Cox M, Diamond I.
Incidence of drug and solvent abuse in normal fourth and fifth year comprehensive school children - some socio-behavioural characteristics.
Brit J Soc Work 1986; 16: 341-351

Prockop L.
Neurotoxic volatile substances.
Neurology 1979; 29: 862-865

Raczka RA.
The effects of solvent abuse: an investigation into the neuropsychological functioning of a group of solvent abusers. ·
Unpublished MSc (Clinical psychology) Dissertation, 1983

Ramsey AW.
Solvent abuse: An educational perspective.
Hum Toxicol 1982; 1: 265-270

Reed BJ, May PA.
Inhalant abuse and juvenile delinquency: a control study in Alberquerque, New Mexico.
Int J Addict 1984; 19: 789-803

Reitan RM.
An investigation of the validity of Halstead's methods of biological intelligence.
Arch Neurol Psychiat 1955; 73: 28-35

Ron MA.
Brain damage in chronic alcoholism: A neuropathological, neuroradiological and psychological review.
Psychol Med 1977; 7: 103-112

Ron MA.
The alcoholic brain: CT scan and psychological findings.
Psychol Med 1983; Monog Suppl 3

Ron MA.
Volatile substance abuse: A review of possible long-term neurological, intellectual and psychiatric sequelae
Brit J Psychiat 1986; 148: 235-246

Rutter M.
A Children's behaviour questionnaire for completion by teachers: Preliminary findings.
J Child Psychol Psychiat 1967; 8: 1-11

Rutter M.
Changing Youth in a Changing Society.
Nuffield Provincial Hospitals Trust: London, 1979

Rutter M, Giller H.
Juvenile Delinquency: Trends and Perspectives.
Pengiun Books: Harmondsworth, Middlesex, 1983

Rutter O, Chadwick O.
Neurobehavioural associations and syndromes of "minimal brain dysfunction".
In Rose FC (Ed), Clinical Neuroepidemiology.
Pitman Medical: London, 1980

Rutter M, Graham P, Chadwick O, Yule W.
Adolescent turmoil: Fact or fiction?
J Child Psychol Psychiat 1976; 17: 35-36

Rutter M, Graham P, Yule W.
A Neuropsychiatric Study in Childhood.
Clinics in Developmental Medicine Nos 35-36,
Spastics International Medical Publications/Heinemann Medical Books: London, 1970

Rutter M, Tizard J, Whitmore K.
Education, health and behaviour.
Longman: London, 1970

Schaffer S.
Substance abuse among Alabama adolescents.
Alabama J Med Sci 1984; 31: 259-261

Schikler KN, Laine EE, Seitz K, Collins WM.
Solvent abuse associated pulmonary abnormalities.
Adv Alcohol Subst Abuse 1984; 3: 75-81

Schikler KN, Seitz K, Rice JF, Strader T.
Solvent abuse associated cortical atrophy.
J Adolesc Health Care 1982; 3: 37-39

Skuse D, Burrell S.
A review of solvent abusers and their management by a child psychiatric outpatient service.
Human Toxicol 1982; 1: 321-330

Smart RG.
Solvent abuse in North America: Aspects of epidemiology,
prevention and treatment.
J Psychoactive Drugs 1986; 18: 87-96

Smart RG, Fejer D.
Six years of cross-sectional surveys of student drug use in Toronto.
Bull Narcotics 1975; 27: 11-22

Smart RG, Adlaf EM, Goodstadt MS.
Alcohol and other drug use among Ontario students in 1985, and trends since 1977.
Addiction Research Foundation: Toronto, 1985.

Smith M, Delves T, Lansdown R, Clayton B, Graham P.
The effects of lead exposure on urban children:
The Institute of Child Health/Southampton Study
Devel Med Child Neurol 1983; 25: Suppl 47

Sokol J, Robinson JL.
Glue sniffing.
Western Med 1963; 4: 192-3, 196, 214

Stephens RC, Diamond SC, Speciman CR et al.
Sniffing from Suffolk to Syracuse: A report on youthful solvent abuse in New York State.
Presented at the First International Symposium on Voluntary Inhalation of Industrial Solvents, Mexico City, 1976

Sterling JW.
A comparative examination of two modes of intoxication - an exploratory study of glue sniffing.
J Crim Law Criminol Pol Sci 1964; 55: 94-97

Stimson GV.
Epidemiological research on drug use in general populations. In Edwards G, Busch C (Eds), Drug Problems in Britain. Academic Press: London 1981

Stuart P.
Solvents and schoolchildren- knowledge and experimentation among a group of young people aged 11 to 18
Health Educ J 1986; 45: 84-86

Swadi H.
Drug and substance abuse among 3,333 London adolescents.
Brit J Addict 1988; 83: 935-942

Tarter RE.
Psychological deficit in chronic alcoholics: A review.
Int J Addict 1975; 10: 327-368

Taylor HG, Michaels RH, Mazr PM, Bauer RE, Liden CB.
Intellectual, neuropsychological, and achievement outcomes in children six to eight years after recovery from Haemophilus influenza meningitis.
Pediatrics 1984; 74: 198-205

Towfighi J, Gonatas NK, Pleasure D, Cooper HS, McCree L.
Glue sniffer's neuropathy.
Neurology 1976; 26: 238-243

Trites RL, Suh M, Offord D, Nieman G, Preston D.
Neuropsychologic and psychosocial antecedents and chronic effects of prolonged use of solvent and metamphetamine.
Psychiat J Univ Ottawa 1976; 1: 14-20.

Tsushima WT, Towne WS.
Effects of paint sniffing on neuropsychological test performance.
J Abnorm Psychol 1977; 86: 402-407

Tsushima WT, Wedding D.
A comparison of the Halstead-Reitain neuropsychological battery and computerized tomography in the identification of brain disorder.
J Nerv Ment Dis 1979; 167: 704-707

Waldron HA.
Solvents and the brain.
Brit J Ind Med 1986; 43: 73-74

Watson JM.
Solvent abuse: The adolescent epidemic?
Croom Helm: London, 1986

Watson JM.
Clinical and laboratory investigations in 132 cases of solvent abuse.
Med Sci Law 1978; 18: 40-43

92

Watson JM.
Morbidity and mortality statistics on solvent abuse.
Med Sci Law 1979; 19: 246-252

Wechsler D.
The Measurement of Adult Intelligence.
3rd Edition Williams and Wilkins: Baltimore, 1944

Wechsler D.
Wechsler Intelligence Scale for Children-Revised.
The Psychological Corporation: New York, 1974

Wert RC, Raulin ML.
The chronic cerebral effects of cannabis use:
I Methodological issues and neurological findings.
Int J Addict 1986; 21: 605-628 (a)

Wert RC, Raulin ML.
The chronic cerebral effects of cannabis use:
II Psychological findings and conclusions
Int J Addict 1986; 21: 629-642 (b)

Whitehead PC
The incidence of drug use among Halifax adolescents.
Brit J Addict 1970; 65 159-165

Williams M.
The Thatcher generation.
New Soc 1986; 21 Feb: 312-315

Winneke G.
Neurobehavioural and neuropsychological effects of lead.
In Rutter M, Russell Jones R (Eds) Lead Versus health.
Wiley, Chichester, 1983

Yancy WS, Nader PR, Burnham KL.
Drug use and attitudes of high school students.
Pediat 1972; 50: 739-745

Yule W.
Diagnosis: Developmental psychological assessment.
Adv Biol Psychiat 1978; 1: 35-54

Zur J, Yule W.
Chronic solvent abuse: I Cognitive sequelae.
Child: Health Care Devel (1990a; 16: 1-20)

Zur J, Yule W.
Chronic solvent abuse: II Relationship with depression.
Child: Health Care Devel (1990b; 21-34)

Tables

Table 1

VOLATILE COMPONENTS OF ABUSED PRODUCTS

Product	Volatile component
Adhesives	
Contact adhesives	Toluene mostly
PVC cement	Trichloroethylene
Balsa wood cement	Ethyl acetate mostly
Cycle tyre repair	Toluene & xylene
Latex	White spirit
Super glue	No significant volatiles
Aerosols	
Air freshener	Propellant 11 & 12
Deodorants, anti-perspirants	Propellant 11 & 12
Fly spray	Propellant 11 & 12 & butane
Hair lacquer	Propellant 11 & 12
Local analgestic spray	Propellant 11 & 12
Paint	Propellant 11 & 12 & esters
Anaesthetic agents	
Liquid	Halothane
Gaseous	Nitrous oxide
Local	Propellant 11 & 12
Cosmetics (non aerosol)	
Nail varnish remover	Acetone & esters
Dry cleaning agents	Tetrachloroethylene
Degreasing agents	1,1,1-trichloroethane trichloroethylene
Fire extinguishers	Bromochlorodifluoromethane Propellant 11 & 12
Fuel gases	
Cigarette lighter refills	n-butane & iso-butane
Butane	n-butane & iso-butane
Propane	Propane & butane isomers
Paint stripper	Dichloromethane Toluene
Spot removers & dry cleaners	
General	1,1,1-trichloroethane Tetrachloroethylene Trichloroethylene
Tar remover	White Spirit
Typewriter correcting fluid & thinners	1,1,1-trichloroethane

96

Table 2

PHYSICAL PROPERTIES AND OCCUPATIONAL
EXPOSURE LEVELS OF VOLATILE SUBSTANCES

Compound	BPt	OEL
Halogenated compunds		
Bromochlorodifluoromethane (1)	-4	-
Dichlorodifluoromethane (2)	-30	1000
Trichlorofluoromethane (3)	24	1000
Dichloromethane	40	200
1,1,1-Trichloroethane	74	350
Trichloroethylene	87	100
Tetrachloroethylene	121	100
Bromochlorotrifluoroethane (4)	50	-
Hydrocarbons		
Aromatic		
Toluene	111	100
Xylene	140	100
Aliphatic		
Propane (5)	-42	-
n-Butane (5)	-1	-
iso-butane (5)	-12	-
n-Hexane	69	100
Mixed		
Petrol	60-2-4	-
White spirit	150-200	100
Others		
Esters		
Ethyl acetate	77	400
Ketones		
Acetone	57	1000
Butan-2-one	80	200
Permanent gasses		
Nitrous oxide	-88	-

Notes:
Bpt. Boiling point at atmospheric pressure in degrees Celsius.
OEL. Occupational Exposure Limit in parts per million.
1. BCF
2. Propellant 12
3. Propellant 11
4. Halothane
5. Components of liquefied petroleum gas (LPG)
OEL=1000ppm.

Table 3

POPULATION SURVEYED AND QUESTIONNAIRE RETURN AT EACH OF THE SCHOOLS

School	Area	Sex	School years surveyed	Number on register	Parental refusals No.	%	Absentees No.	%	Completed questionnaires	%
1	C	Mixed	3,4,5	374	34	9.1	71	19.0	235	62.8
2	B	Mixed	3,4,5	648	28	4.3	68	10.5	504	77.8
3	B	Mixed	3,4,5	415	39	9.4	59	14.2	302	72.3
4	A	Girls	3,4,5	556	22	4.0	69	12.4	398	71.6
5	A	Boys	4,5	519	43	8.3	50	9.6	348	67.0
6	A	Mixed	3,4,5	482	59	12.2	105	21.8	280	58.1
7	B	Mixed	3,4,5	748	44	5.9	Not known		478	63.9
8	B	Mixed	3,4,5	623	58	9.3	161	25.8	403	64.7
9	C	Girls	3,4,5	563	197	35.0	82	14.6	303	53.8
10	A	Girls	3,4,5	521	82	15.7	90	17.3	360	69.1
11	C	Boys	3,4	383	82	21.4	61	15.9	251	65.5
12	B	Boys	4,5	349	0	0.0	75	21.5	268	76.8
13	A	Girls	3,4	411	65	15.8	79	19.2	277	67.4
14	B	Mixed	3,4,5	571	52	9.1	154	27.0	375	65.7
15	B	Girls	4	159	11	6.9	25	15.7	115	72.3
16	B	Boys	4	163	9	5.5	31	19.0	117	71.8
ALL				7485	825	11.0	1180	15.8	5014	67.0

98

Table 4

COMPOUNDS THAT COULD BE IDENTIFIED
ON COARSE SCREEN BY PETRA

Channel	m/z Ratio	Compound
1	46	Carbon dioxide
2	85	Bromochlorodifluoromethane (BCF) Chloroform Halon 12 Halon 114
3	91	Toluene, ? Petrol
4	61	1,1,1-Trichloroethane
5	101	Halon 11 Halon 12 Halon 114 1,1,1-Trichloroethane
6	164	Tetrachloroethylene
7	97	1,1,1-Trichloroethane Trichloroethane
8	58	Acetone Butane Isobutane

Table 5

COMPARABILITY OF CASES AND CONTROLS
ON MATCHING VARIABLES

		Controls (n=105)		Solvent abusers (n=105)	
		n	%	n	%
School year (at initial interview assessment)	3rd	20	19.0	20	19.0
	4th	61	58.1	61	58.1
	5th	24	22.9	24	22.9
Sex	Boys	44	41.9	44	41.9
	Girls	61	58.1	6	58.1
School	1	6	5.7	3	5.7
	2	7	6.6	8	7.6
	3	9	8.6	9	8.6
	4	1	0.9	1	0.9
	5	6	5.7	7	6.6
	6	10	9.5	10	9.5
	7	3	2.9	3	2.9
	8	10	9.5	7	6.6
	9	10	9.5	10	9.5
	10	8	7.6	10	9.5
	11	16	15.2	16	15.2
	12	3	2.9	4	3.8
	13	10	9.5	11	10.5
	14	4	3.8	4	3.8
	15	2	1.9	2	1.9
	16	0	1.0	0	0.0

Table 6

PREVALENCE OF SOLVENT ABUSE (EVER) BY SEX IN CHILDREN ATTENDING SINGLE-SEX AND CO-EDUCATIONAL SCHOOLS

	Boys only schools (n=3)				Girls only school (n=4)				Coeducational schools (n=6)			
	N	n	%	(95% C.I.)	N	n	%	(95% C.I.)	N	n	%	(95% C.I.)
Boys	733	8	1.1	(0.3-1.8)	-	-	-	-	1222	47	3.8	(2.7-4.9)
Girls	-	-			1150	51	4.4	(3.2-5.6)	1116	44	3.9	(2.8-5.1)

N = sample size.
n = solvent abusers.
CI = confidence intervals.

Table 7

**PREVALENCE OF SOLVENT ABUSE (EVER)
BY SCHOOL YEAR AND SEX IN CHILDREN ATTENDING
CO-EDUCATIONAL SCHOOLS**

School year	Boys			Girls			Total		
	N	n	%	N	n	%	N	n	%
3rd	464	8	1.7	388	13	3.3	852	21	2.5
4th	403	20	5.0	381	20	5.2	784	40	5.1
5th	345	18	5.2	330	11	3.3	675	29	4.3
All	1212	46	3.8	1099	44	4.0	2311	90	3.9

b) 95% Confidence intervals

School year	Boys		Girls		Total	
	%	(95% C.I.)	%	(95% C.I.)	%	(95% C.I.)
3rd	1.7	0.5 - 2.9	3.3	1.6 - 5.1	2.5	1.4 - 3.5
4th	5.0	2.8 - 7.1	5.2	3.0 - 7.5	5.1	3.6 - 6.6
5th	5.2	2.9 - 7.6	3.3	1.4 - 5.3	4.3	2.8 - 5.8
All	3.8	2.7 - 4.9	4.0	2.8 - 5.2	3.9	3.1 - 4.7

Table 8
FREQUENCY OF SOLVENT ABUSE (EVER) BY SCHOOL YEAR

	3rd year (n=1275)			4th year (n=1699)			5th year (n=1218)			Total (n=4192)		
	n	Prev. %	Rel. Freq. %	n	Prev. %	Rel. Freq. %	n	Prev. %	Rel. Freq. %	n	Prev. %	Rel. Freq. %
1 - 2 Times	18	1.4	56.2	32	1.9	42.7	16	1.3	47.1	66	1.6	47.5
3 - 4 Times	4	0.3	13.3	13	0.8	17.3	5	0.4	14.7	22	0.5	15.8
5 - 9 Times	4	0.3	13.3	14	0.8	18.7	4	0.3	11.8	22	0.5	15.8
10 - 30 Times	2	0.2	6.7	12	0.7	16.0	4	0.3	11.8	18	0.4	12.9
> 30 Times	2	0.2	6.7	4	0.2	5.3	5	0.4	14.7	11	0.3	7.9
Not known	2			3			4			9		
	32	2.5	100.0	78	4.6	100.0	38	3.1	100.0	148	3.5	100.0

Table 9

FREQUENCY OF SOLVENT ABUSE

	Boys (n=1955)			Girls (n=2260)			Total (n=4215)		
	n	Prev. %	Rel. Freq. %	n	Prev. %	Rel. Freq. %	n	Prev. %	Rel. Freq. %
1 - 2 Times	22	1.1	44.0	43	1.9	48.3	65	1.5	46.8
3 - 4 Times	7	0.4	14.0	15	0.7	16.8	22	0.5	15.8
5 - 9 Times	9	0.5	18.0	14	0.6	15.7	23	0.5	16.5
10 - 30 Times	6	0.3	12.0	12	0.5	13.5	18	0.4	12.9
> 30 Times	6	0.3	12.0	5	0.2	5.6	11	0.3	7.9
Not known	5			4			9		
	55	2.8	100.0	93	4.1	100.0	148	3.5	100.0

Table 10

TYPES OF PRODUCT ABUSED BY SCHOOL YEAR

Type of product abused	3rd year (n=1275)			4th year (n=1699)			5th year (n=1218)			Total (n=4192)		
	n	Prev. %	Rel. Freq. %	n	Prev. %	Rel. Freq. %	n	Prev. %	Rel. Freq. %	n	Prev. %	Rel. Freq. %
TCFs	18	1.4	54.5	52	3.1	65.8	25	2.0	65.8	95	2.3	63.3
Gas	11	0.9	33.3	30	1.8	38.0	12	1.0	31.6	53	1.3	35.3
Glue	9	0.7	27.3	23	1.3	29.1	11	0.9	28.9	43	1.0	28.7
DCFs&DGAs	0	0.0	0.0	3	0.2	3.7	3	0.2	7.9	6	0.1	4.0
Petrol	2	0.2	6.1	3	0.2	3.7	0	0.0	0.0	5	0.1	3.3
Amyl nitrate	0	0.0	0.0	3	0.2	3.7	2	0.2	5.3	5	0.1	3.3
Paints etc.	0	0.0	0.0	1	0.1	1.3	0	0.0	0.0	1	0.0	0.7
Aerosols	0	0.0	0.0	1	0.1	1.3	0	0.0	0.0	1	0.0	0.7
Other	0	0.0	0.0	1	0.1	1.3	0	0.0	0.0	1	0.0	0.7
No. of Cases	33			79			38			150		

TCFs: Typewriter correction fluids
Paints: Paint, white spirit, turpentine
DCFs & DGAs: Dry cleaning fluids and degreasing agents

Table 11

TYPES OF PRODUCT ABUSED BY SEX

Type of product abused	Boys (n=1955)			Girls (n=2260)			Total (n=4215)		
	n	Prev. %	Rel. Freq. %	n	Prev. %	Rel. Freq. %	n	Prev. %	Rel. Freq. %
TCFs	32	1.6	57.1	64	2.8	68.1	96	2.3	64.0
Gas	22	1.1	39.3	32	1.4	34.0	54	1.3	36.0
Glue	27	1.4	48.2	16	0.7	17.0	43	1.0	28.7
DCFs&DGAs	4	0.2	7.1	3	0.3	3.2	7	0.2	4.7
Petrol	5	0.3	8.9	0	0.0	0.0	5	0.1	3.3
Amyl nitrite	0	0.0	0.0	5	0.2	5.3	5	0.1	3.3
Paints etc.	0	0.0	0.0	1	0.0	1.1	1	0.0	0.7
Aerosols	1	0.0	1.8	0	0.0	0.0	1	0.0	0.7
Other	1	0.0	1.8	0	0.0	0.0	1	0.0	1.7
No. of Cases	56			94			150		

TCFS   : Typewriter correction fluids
Paints etc.   : Paint, white spirtit, turpentine
DCFs & DGAs : Dry-cleaning fluids and degreasing agents

Table 12

NUMBER OF DIFFERENT TYPES OF PRODUCT ABUSED PER CASE BY SCHOOL YEAR

Number of different types of product abused	3rd year (n=1275)			4th year (n=1699)			5th year (n=1218)			Total (n=4192)		
	n	Prev. %	Rel. Freq. %	n	Prev. %	Rel. Freq. %	n	Prev. %	Rel. Freq. %	n	Prev. %	Rel. Freq. %
One	20	1.6	69.0	40	2.3	54.8	16	1.3	48.5	76	1.8	52.4
Two	7	0.5	24.1	25	1.5	34.2	11	0.9	33.3	43	1.0	31.8
Three	1	0.1	3.4	5	0.3	6.8	6	0.5	18.1	12	0.3	8.9
Four	1	0.1	3.4	2	0.1	2.7	0	0.0	0.0	3	0.1	2.2
Five	0	0.0	0.0	0	0.0	0.0	0	0.0	0.0	0	0.0	0.0
Six	0	0.0	0.0	0	0.0	0.0	0	0.0	0.0	1	0.0	0.7
Not known	4			6			5			15		
Total	33	2.6	100.0	38	3.1	100.0	38	3.1	100.0	150	3.6	100.0

Table 13

NUMBER OF DIFFERENT TYPES OF PRODUCT ABUSED
PER CASE BY SEX

Number of different types of product abused	Boys (n = 1955)			Girls (n = 2260)			Total (n = 4215)		
	n	Prev. %	Rel. Freq. %	n	Prev. %	Rel. Freq. %	n	Prev. %	Rel. Freq. %
One	22	1.1	44.9	54	2.4	62.1	76	1.8	55.9
Two	15	0.8	30.6	28	1.2	32.2	43	1.0	31.6
Three	8	0.4	16.3	5	0.2	5.7	13	0.3	9.6
Four	3	0.1	6.1	0	0.0	0.0	3	0.1	2.2
Five	0	0.0	0.0	0	0.0	0.0	0	0.0	0.0
Six	1	0.0	2.0	0	0.0	0.0	1	0.0	0.7
Not known	7			7			14		
Total	56	2.8	100.0	94	4.2	100.0	150	3.6	100.0

Table 14

AGREEMENT BETWEEN QUESTIONNAIRE AND INTERVIEW RESPONSES TO QUESTIONS RELATING TO SOLVENT ABUSE (EVER)

| | Questionnaire response | | |
| | Solvent abuse (ever) | | |
	No	Yes	Total
Interview response			
No	113	20	133
Yes, but not intoxicated	0	7	7
Yes, to intoxication	0	106[a]	106
Total	113	133	

[a] Includes one child who gave an ambiguous response on the questionnaire.

Table 15

CASES WHO WERE POSITIVE ON TOXICOLOGICAL EXAMINATION

Interview findings		Toxicological examination	
Case or Control	Product last abused	Substance identified	Concentration (ppm)
Case	Typewriter correction fluid	1,1,1-Trichloroethane	46
Case	Typewriter correction fluid	1,1,1-Trichloroethane	5.9
Case	Typewriter correction fluid	1,1,1-Trichloroethane	3.5
Case	Typewriter correction fluid	1,1,1-Trichloroethane	1.1
Case	Typewriter correction fluid	1,1,1-Trichloroethane	1.1
Case	Typewriter correction fluid	1,1,1-Trichloroethane	0.6
Case	Petrol	Toluene	0.13
Control	None	Toluene	0.9

Table 16

RESULTS OF TOXICOLOGICAL EXAMINATION IN RELATION TO TIME SINCE SOLVENTS WERE LAST ABUSED (INTERVIEW FINDINGS)

Interview findings Time since last abused solvents	Toxicological examination	
	Positive (n =7)	Negative (n = 93)
1 day	0	2
2-3 days	2	1
4-7 days	0	2
> 1 week to 4 weeks	2	9
> 4 weeks to 6 months	1	32
> 6 months to 1 year	2	23
> 1 year to 2 years	0	16
> 2 years	0	6

Table 17

**FREQUENCY OF SOLVENT ABUSE IN QUESTIONNAIRE-
IDENTIFIED AND INTERVIEW-CONFIRMED CASES**

Boroughs	Questionnaire identified cases*				Interview-confirmed cases**	
	A & B		A, B & C		A, B & C	
	n	%	n	%	n	%
1 - 2 Times	66	47.5	92	47.2	35	33.9
3 - 4 Times	22	15.8	27	13.8	15	14.6
5 - 9 Times	22	15.8	32	16.4	16	15.5
10 - 30 Times	18	12.9	26	13.3	17	16.5
> 30 Times	11	7.9	18	9.2	20	19.4
Not known	12		13		2	
Total	151	100.0	208	100.0	105	100.0

* Questionnaire response

** Interview response

Table 18

TYPE OF PRODUCT ABUSED IN QUESTIONNAIRE-IDENTIFIED AND INTERVIEW-CONFIRMED CASES

Boroughs	Questionnaire-Identified Cases*				Interview-Confirmed Cases**	
	A and B (n=151)		A, B and C (n = 208)		A, B and C (n = 105)	
	n	%	n	%	n	%
Typewriter correcting fluid	95	63.3	134	64.4	80	76.2
Gas lighter fuel/butane gas	53	35.3	65	31.2	29	27.6
Glue	43	28.7	61	29.3	32	30.5
Dry cleaning fluids/ degreasing agents	6	4.0	8	3.8	7	6.7
Petrol	5	3.3	7	3.4	2	1.9
Amyl nitrite	5	3.3	6	2.9	5	4.8
Paints etc	1	0.7	3	1.4	1	0.9
Aerosols	1	0.7	3	1.4	1	0.9
Paint stripper	0	0.0	0	0.0	2	1.9
Other	1	0.7	2	1.0	1	0.9

*   Questionnaire response
**   Interview response

Table 19

**NUMBER OF DIFFERENT TYPES OF PRODUCTS ABUSED PER
CASE IN QUESTIONNAIRE-IDENTIFIED AND
INTERVIEW-CONFIRMED CASES**

Number of different products abused	Questionnaire-identified sample of cases*				Interview confirmed sample of cases**	
Boroughs	**A and B**		**A, B and C**		**A, B and C**	
	n	**%**	**n**	**%**	**n**	**%**
One	76	55.7	106	57.6	66	64.1
Two	43	31.6	54	29.3	23	22.3
Three	13	9.6	16	8.7	10	9.7
Four	3	2.2	7	3.8	3	2.9
Five	0	0.0	0	0.0	1	1.0
Six	1	0.7	1	0.5	0	0.0
Not known	15			24	2	
Total	151	100.0	208	100.0	105	100.0

*   Questionnaire response
**   Interview response

Table 20

INITIAL AND MOST RECENT EPISODES OF SOLVENT ABUSE*
IN INTERVIEW-CONFIRMED CASES

Time since	Initial episode		Most recent episode	
	n	%	n	%
< 1 week ago	0	0.0	8	7.8
1 week - 1 month ago	3	3.3	11	10.7
1-6 months ago	23	25.0	33	32.0
6-12 months ago	25	27.2	26	25.2
1-2 years ago	25	27.2	18	17.5
> 2 years ago	16	17.4	7	6.8
Not known	13		2	
Total	105	100.0	105	100.0

* Interview response

Table 21

SOCIAL CONTEXT AND PREFERRED PLACE OF SNIFFING*
IN INTERVIEW-CONFIRMED CASES **

Social context	n	%
Alone	2	4.2
Sometimes with others, sometimes alone	8	17.0
With others	37	78.7
Not known	6	
Total	53	100.0

Preferred place	n	%
Usually at home	2	4.3
Usuallly at friend's home	4	8.7
Usually at school	2	4.3
Usually in public space (e.g. cemetry, park etc)	38	82.6
Not known	7	
Total	53	100.0

*   Interview responses
**   Data obtained only on cases who sniffed five or more times.

Table 22

AGE, SEX AND ETHNIC BACKGROUND

	Controls (n=105)		Solvent abusers (n=105)	
Age				
In months (mean and SD)	179.6	8.9	180.3	8.6
	(No	%)	(No	%)
In years				
13	12	11.4	8	7.6
14	36	34.3	39	37.1
15	50	47.6	44	41.9
16	7	6.7	14	13.3
Sex				
Boys	44	41.9	44	41.9
Girls	61	58.1	61	58.1
Ethnic background			*	
White	79	75.2	99	94.3
Afro-Caribbean	21	20.0	4	3.8
Indian Subcontinent	5	4.8	2	1.9

* $p < 0.001$

Table 23

SOCIAL AND FAMILY FACTORS AND HOUSING

	Controls (n=105)		Solvent abusers (n=105)		
	n	%	n	%	P
Not living with both 'natural' parents (Q)	36	34.3	43	41.3	NS
3 or more sibs (I/V)	27	25.7	42	40.0	*
Accommodation owned by family or paying mortgage (Q)	63	60.0	49	47.6	NS
Occupational status of main breadwinner (I/V)					NS
I, II, III Non-manual	36	37.1	23	28.0	
III Manual	41	42.3	44	53.6	
IV, V	20	20.6	15	18.3	
Employment status of main breadwinner (I/V)					**
Unemployed	3	3.0	13	13.7	

(Q)   : Questionnaire data
(I/V) : Interview data

*   p<0.05
**   p<0.01

Table 24

GENERAL HEALTH AND ACCIDENTS

	Controls (n=105) %		Solvent abusers (n=105) %		Signif.
Ever missed school for more than a month because of illness (I/V)	9	8.6	14	13.5	NS
4 or more days off school during past month because of illness (Q)	28	26.7	34	32.4	NS
Currently taking prescribed medicines (I/V)	13	12.4	14	13.3	NS
Number of accidents (ever) requiring hospital admission (I/V)					
0	89	84.8	79	75.2	NS
1	15	14.3	19	18.1	
2 or more	1	0.9	7	6.7	
Number of accidents (ever) requiring hospital treatment (I/V)					
0	42	40.0	30	29.7	NS
1 - 2	51	48.6	53	52.5	
3 or more	12	11.4	18	17.8	

	Mean (SD)	Mean (SD)	
Height (cms) NS	164.9 (8.1)	163.6 (8.1)	

(Q)   : Questionnaire data
(I/V) : Interview data

Table 25

ACCIDENTS BY SEX BY GROUP

		Controls			Solvent abusers		
		Boys (n=44)		**Girls (n=61)**	**Boys (n=44)**		**Girls (n=61)**
		n	**%**	**n**	**%**	**n**	**%**	**n**	**%**

Number of accidents
(ever) requiring
hospital admission:

0	37(84.1)	52 (85.2)	32(72.7)	4 (77.8)
1	7(15.9)	8 (13.1)NS	7(15.9)	12 (19.7) NS
2 +	0(0.0)	1 (1.6)	5(11.4)	2 (3.3)

Number of accidents
(ever) requiring
hospital treatment:

0	11(25.0)	31 (50.8)	10(24.4)	20 (33.3)
1 -2	21(47.7)	30(49.2)*	21(51.2)	32 (53.3) NS
3 +	12(27.3)	0 (0.0)	10(24.4)	8 (13.3)

* p<0.001

Table 26

RESPIRATORY HEALTH AND ALLERGIES

	Controls (n=105)		Solvent abusers (n=105)		
	n	%	n	%	
Illnesses during past 12 months (Q)					
Asthma or wheeziness	20	19.0	23	21.9	NS
Bronchitis or pneumonia	3	2.9	5	4.8	NS
Hayfever	28	13.3	21	20.0	NS
Eczema	6	5.7	11	10.5	NS
Uses aerosol inhaler (I/V)	7	6.7	5	4.8	NS
Usually cough first thing in the morning (Q)	10	9.5	45	43.7	***
Usually cough during day or at night (Q)	31	29.5	62	59.6	***
Tend to get short of breath (Q)	23	21.9	55	52.4	***

Lung Function Tests	Mean (SD)	Mean (SD)	
Vital Capacity	3.41 (0.82)	3.45 (0.75)	NS
FEV^1	2.97 (0.67)	3.06 (0.63)	NS
Peak Flow	442.8 (61.1)	440.1 (62.8)	NS

(Q):Questionnaire data
(I/V):Interview data

*** p<0.001

Table 27
CIGARETTE SMOKING

	Controls (n=105)		Solvent Abusers (n=105)		
	n	%	n	%	
History of Smoking (I/V)					***
Never smoked	34	32.4	1	0.9	
Only once or twice ever	32	30.5	8	7.6	
Used to occasionally	12	11.4	7	6.7	
Used to regularly	7	6.7	7	6.7	
Currently smokes	20	19.0	82	78.1	
Last Smoked					***
Earlier today (I/V)	13	12.4	67	65.0	
Yesterday	3	2.9	12	11.6	
2-7 days ago	2	1.9	4	3.9	
1 week - 1 month ago	3	2.9	2	1.9	
> 1 < 12 months ago	17	16.2	5	4.8	
> 1 year ago	26	24.8	12	11.6	
Never	41	39.0	1	1.0	
Frequency of Smoking Now (I/V):					***
None	86	81.9	23	21.9	
1 or 2 per day or less	4	3.8	10	9.5	
> 2 < 10 per day	12	11.4	46	43.8	
> 10 < 20 per day	3	2.9	24	22.9	
> 20 per day	0	0.0	2	1.9	
Father Smokes (Q)	45	50.0	58	63.7	NS
Mother Smokes (Q)	39	37.9	55	56.7	*

I/V   Interview data
Questionnaire data

*   P< 0.05
**   P< 0.01
***   P< 0.001

Table 28

ALCOHOL (INTERVIEW DATA)

	Controls (n=105)		Solvent abusers (n=105)		
	n	%	n	%	
Last had a drink					***
Yesterday	4	3.8	13	12.5	
2 - 4 days ago	18	17.1	31	29.8	
> 4 < 7 days ago	14	13.3	15	14.4	
> 7 days < 1 month ago	24	22.9	28	26.9	
> 1 < 12 months ago	33	31.4	14	13.5	
> 1 year ago	3	2.9	1	1.0	
Never	9	8.6	2	1.9	
Frequency of drinking					***
Not at all	9	8.6	2	2.0	
Special occasions only	35	33.6	9	9.0	
< once a week	40	38.5	44	44.0	
Once or twice a week	20	19.2	31	31.0	
> once or twice a week	0	0.0	14	14.0	
Every day	0	0.0	0	0.0	
Last occasion drunk					***
Yesterday	0	0.0	1	1.0	
2 - 4 days ago	1	1.0	12	12.1	
> 4 < 7 days ago	3	2.9	7	7.1	
> 7 days < 1 month ago	6	5.9	24	24.2	
> 1 < 12 months ago	25	24.5	32	32.3	
> 1 year ago	7	6.9	4	4.0	
Never	60	58.8	19	19.2	
Frequency of drunkeness					***
Never	60	57.7	20	20.6	
Once or twice ever	24	23.1	14	14.4	
3 - 4 times ever	8	7.7	9	9.3	
Once a month or less	9	8.6	38	39.2	
< once a week	2	1.9	11	11.3	
1 - 2 times per week	1	1.0	3	3.1	
> 1 - 2 times per week	0	0.0	2	2.1	

*** $P < 0.001$

Table 29

BEHAVIORAL AND EMOTIONAL
ASPECTS OF HEALTH (BOYS)

	Controls (n=44)		Solvent abusers (n=44)		Signif	Odds ratio
	n	%	n	%		
Sleeping difficulties	3	6.8	6	13.9	NS	2.0
Not eating	2	4.5	4	9.1	NS	2.0
Stomach aches	3	6.8	5	11.6	NS	1.7
Headaches	7	16.3	8	19.5	NS	1.2
Tense/nervous	3	7.0	3	7.3	NS	1.0
Poor concentration	8	18.2	16	37.2	*	2.0
Worrying	6	13.6	5	11.4	NS	0.8
Teased/bullied	4	9.1	3	7.1	NS	0.8
Involved in fights	0	0.0	12	27.9	***	<12.3
Stealing	1	2.3	13	30.2	**	13.3
Destructive	0	0.0	7	16.3	*	< 7.2
Truancy	2	4.6	11	25.0	*	5.4
Misery	3	6.8	1	2.3	NS	0.3
Loneliness	1	2.3	2	4.6	NS	2.0
Worried about health	4	9.1	5	11.4	NS	1.2
	Mean	(SD)	Mean	(SD)		
Total score	12.2	(6.5)	19.0	(6.9)	***	
Mean score per item	1.4	(1.7)	2.2	(1.3)	*	

*   P < 0.05
**   P < 0.01
*** P < 0.001

Table 30

BEHAVIORAL AND EMOTIONAL
ASPECTS OF HEALTH (GIRLS)

	Controls (n=61)		Solvent abusers (n=61)		Signif	Odds ratio
	n	%	n	%		
Sleeping difficulties	10	16.7	10	16.4	NS	1.0
Not eating	11	18.0	24	39.3	**	2.2
Stomach aches	7	11.5	20	33.3	**	2.9
Headaches	15	25.0	20	32.8	NS	1.3
Tense/nervous	7	11.5	12	20.0	NS	1.7
Poor concentration	10	16.4	27	44.3	*	2.7
Worrying	9	15.0	22	36.1	*	2.4
Teased/bullied	0	0.0	3	4.9	NS	> 3.0
Involved in fights	1	1.6	7	11.5	NS	7.0
Stealing	0	0.0	2	3.3	NS	> 2.0
Destructive	0	0.0	1	1.7	NS	> 1.0
Truancy	2	3.3	15	24.6	*	7.5
Misery	8	13.1	17	27.9	*	2.1
Loneliness	5	8.2	13	21.3	*	2.6
Worried about health	4	6.7	10	16.4	NS	2.5
	Mean	(SD)	Mean	(SD)		
Total score	14.8	(7.0)	21.5	(6.4)	***	
Mean score per item	2.1	(1.6)	2.9	(1.5)	*	

*   P < 0.05
**   P < 0.01
***   P < 0.001

Table 31

BEHAVIORAL AND EMOTIONAL ASPECTS OF HEALTH (BOYS) IN SOLVENT ABUSERS AND QUESTIONNAIRE CONTROLS WITH TOTAL SCORES OF 14 OR MORE

	Controls (n=731)		Solvent abusers (n=44)		Odds ratio
Sleeping difficulties	93	(12.7%)	6	(13.9%)	1.1
Not eating	63	(8.6%)	4	(9.1%)	1.0
Stomach aches	84	(11.5%)	5	(11.6%)	1.0
Headaches	147	(20.1%)	8	(19.5%)	1.0
Tense/nervous	77	(10.5%)	3	(7.3%)	0.7
Poor concentration	150	(20.5%)	16	(37.2%)	1.8
Worrying	103	(14.1%)	5	(11.4%)	0.8
Teased/bullied	102	(14.0%)	3	(7.1%)	0.5
Involved in fights	77	(10.5%)	12	(27.9%)	2.6
Stealing	35	(4.8%)	13	(30.2%)	6.3
Destructive	29	(4.0%)	7	(16.3%)	4.1
Truancy	48	(6.6%)	11	(25.0%)	3.8
Misery	99	(13.5%)	1	(2.3%)	0.2
Loneliness	58	(7.9%)	2	(4.6%)	0.6
Worried about health	70	(9.6%)	5	(11.4%)	1.2
	Mean	(SD)	Mean	(SD)	Sig
Total score	18.9	(4.2)	19.0	(6.9)	NS

Table 32

BEHAVIORAL AND EMOTIONAL ASPECTS OF HEALTH (GIRLS) IN SOLVENT ABUSERS AND QUESTIONNAIRE CONTROLS WITH TOTAL SCORES OF 17 OR MORE

	Controls (n=859)		Solvent abusers (n=61)		Odds ratio
Sleeping difficulties	184	(21.4%)	10	(16.4%)	0.8
Not eating	220	(25.6%)	24	(39.3%)	1.5
Stomach aches	252	(29.3%)	20	(33.3%)	1.1
Headaches	291	(33.9%)	20	(32.8%)	1.0
Tense/nervous	190	(22.1%)	12	(20.0%)	0.9
Poor concentration	255	(29.7%)	27	(44.3%)	1.5
Worrying	280	(32.6%)	22	(36.1%)	1.1
Teased/bullied	49	(5.7%)	3	(4.9%)	0.9
Involved in fights	41	(4.8%)	7	(11.5%)	2.4
Stealing	14	(1.6%)	2	(3.3%)	2.0
Destructive	12	(1.4%)	1	(1.7%)	1.2
Truancy	61	(7.1%)	15	(24.6%)	3.5
Misery	261	(30.4%)	17	(27.9%)	0.9
Loneliness	161	(18.7%)	13	(21.3%)	1.1
Worried about health	138	(16.1%)	10	(16.4%)	1.0
	Mean	(SD)	Mean	(SD)	Sig
Total score	21.6	(4.0)	21.5	(6.4)	NS

Table 33

SCHOOL PERFORMANCE AND ATTENDANCE

	Controls (n=105)		Solvent abusers (n=105)		
	n	%	n	%	
Self-Appraisal					*
Doing well	27	**27.3**	12	**13.5**	
About average	67	**67.7**	60	**67.4**	
Not doing very well	5	**5.0**	17	**19.1**	
Favorite subject					
Maths or English	39	**38.2**	27	**27.5**	NS
P.E.	13	**12.7**	13	**13.3**	NS
Relationships with teachers					**
Reasonably well with most	94	**94.0**	61	**62.2**	
Some problems with most or marked antipathy to a few	4	**4.0**	26	**26.5**	
Marked antipathy to most	2	**2.0**	11	**11.2**	
	Mean	(SD)	Mean	(SD)	
No of half days registered absent (Nov 1984)	4.4	**5.8**	5.0	**5.7**	NS
No of half days registered late (Nov 1984)	1.5	**2.9**	3.1	**4.0**	*

*   P< 0.01

** P< 0.001

Table 34

PSYCHOLOGICAL TEST SCORES OF CASES AND CONTROLS MATCHED FOR ETHNIC BACKGROUND

	Controls (n=80)	Solvent abusers (n=80)	Sig
WISC			
Similarities	12.0 (3.3)	11.1 (3.2)	NS
Vocabulary	10.2 (2.5)	9.4 (2.3)	*
Picture Completion	10.4 (2.6)	10.1 (2.8)	NS
Block Design	12.1 (2.8)	11.4 (2.2)	NS
Verbal IQ (Prorated)	106.9 (16.7)	101.3 (14.7)	*
Performance IQ (Prorated)	109.0 (14.6)	105.2 (14.3)	NS
Full Scale IQ (Prorated)	108.8 (15.1)	103.4 (14.3)	*
EH-3 Reading Quotient	103.9 (12.4)	102.0 (13.1)	NS
Passage recall: Items recalled			
Immediate Presentation	10.5 (3.8)	9.6 (3.3)	NS
Delayed Presentation	10.1 (3.7)	9.0 (3.5)	NS
Speed of information processing			
T-Score	52.3 (8.1)	50.5 (7.0)	NS
Manual dexterity			
Right Hand (Time in Secs)	10.2 (1.1)	10.2 (1.0)	NS
Left Hand (Time in Secs)	11.0 (1.2)	11.0 (1.4)	NS
Vibration sensation threshold			
Thumbe	3.2 (1.8)	3.2 (1.2)	NS
Ankle	7.3 (4.6)	7.1 (2.1)	NS

Table 34 (continued)

PSYCHOLOGICAL TEST SCORES OF CASES AND CONTROLS MATCHED FOR ETHNIC BACKGROUND

	Controls (n=80)	Solvent abusers (n=80)	Sig
Bexley-Maudsley Automated Tests			
Visual discrimination			
Mean RT: Grade 2	5.4 (1.3)	5.7 (1.8)	NS
Mean RT: Grade 4	3.9 (1.1)	4.0 (1.1)	NS
Errors: Grade 2	0.7 (1.2)	1.0 (1.5)	NS
Errors: Grade 4	0.4 (0.9)	0.5 (0.9)	NS
Symbol-digit coding			
Mean RT: 1st 15	1.95 (0.29)	2.02 (0.35)	NS
Mean RT: 2nd 15	1.85 (0.30)	1.93 (0.37)	NS
Mean RT: 3rd 15	1.80 (0.28)	1.85 (0.32)	NS
Mean RT: All 45	1.86 (0.25)	1.94 (0.31)	NS
Mistakes: All 45	1.0	1.0	NS
Reaction time tests			
A) Two choice Mean RT: either hand	0.364 (0.073)	0.373 (0.084)	NS
Left-right errors	2.1 (1.1)	2.3 (2.2)	NS
B) Two Choice with inhibition Mean RT: either hand	0.561 (0.121)	0.595 (0.148)	NS
Failed inhibitory responses	1.2 (1.3)	1.9 (2.0)	*
Finger tapping (Taps per sec)			
Right Hand Index	5.8 (1.4)	6.1 (1.7)	NS
Left Hand Index	5.3 (1.1)	5.0 (1.2)	NS
Right Hand Index/Middle	2.5 (0.8)	2.5 (0.9)	NS
Left Hand Index/Middle	2.2 (0.7)	2.3 (0.7)	NS
Right/Left Hand Index	3.4 (0.8)	3.7 (1.0)	NS
Trail-making (Secs per target)			
1-9	2.5 (1.0)	2.3 (0.5)	NS
1-9 Alternating	3.2 (0.9)	3.1 (0.6)	NS

* $p < 0.05$

Table 35

SUBSIDIARY PSYCHOLOGICAL TEST MEASURES: STANDARD DEVIATIONS OF MEAN (WITHIN-SUBJECT) REACTION TIME RESPONSES IN PAIRS MATCHED FOR ETHNIC BACKGROUND

	Controls (n=80)	Solvent abusers (n=80)	Sig
Bexley-Maudsley Automated Tests			
A) Grade 2:			
s.d. of mean RT (correct Rs)	2.53 (1.18)	2.55 (1.34)	NS
B) Grade 4:			
s.d. of mean RT (correct Rs)	1.69 (0.87)	1.71 (0.85)	NS
Symbol-digit coding			
s.d. of mean RT: 1st 15	0.54 (0.29)	0.59 (0.31)	NS
s.d. of mean RT: 2nd 15	0.53 (0.30)	0.57 (0.30)	NS
s.d. of mean RT: 3rd 15	0.54 (0.29)	0.57 (0.25)	NS
s.d. of mean RT: All 45	0.57 (0.22)	0.61 (0.21)	NS
Reaction time tests			
A) Two choice			
s.d. of mean RT: Left hand	0.085 (0.041)	0.084 (0.041)	NS
s.d. of mean RT: Right hand	0.081 (0.052)	0.075 (0.043)	NS
B) Two choice with inhibition			
s.d. of mean RT: Left hand	0.126 (0.060)	0.139 (0.072)	NS
s.d. of mean RT: Right hand	0.121 (0.057)	0.161 (0.146)	*

* $p < 0.05$

Table 36

MEAN CASE-CONTROL DIFFERENCES IN PSYCHOLOGICAL TEST SCORESAND FREQUENCY OF SOLVENT ABUSE IN PAIRS MATCHED FOR ETHNIC BACKGROUND

	Frequency of Solvent Abuse						
	1-2 Times	3-4 Times	5-9 Times	10-30 Times	> 30 Times	Test for linear trend	
	(n=27)	(n=11)	(n=11)	(n=15)	(n=14)	Sig	Sig
WISC							
Similarities	+ 1.5 (4.8)	- 0.6 (5.6)	+ 1.6 (6.1)	+ 0.2 (3.4)	+ 1.2 (3.3)	NS	NS
Vocabulary	+ 0.8 (3.8)	+ 1.3 (3.5)	+ 1.4 (3.5)	+ 1.1 (3.3)	- 0.4 (3.1)	NS	NS
Picture Completion	+ 0.1 (3.7)	- 0.1 (3.6)	- 0.7 (4.4)	+ 1.3 (2.6)	+ 0.7 (2.9)	NS	NS
Block Design	+ 0.6 (3.7)	- 0.4 (3.8)	+ 1.6 (4.8)	+ 1.3 (4.1)	+ 1.0 (3.8)	NS	NS
Verbal IQ (Prorated)	+ 7.1 (24.3)	+ 2.1 (25.4)	+ 9.4 (25.6)	+ 3.9 (19.2)	+ 2.4 (17.1)	NS	NS
Performance IQ (Prorated)	+ 2.3 (21.8)	- 3.0 (24.2)	+ 4.0 (22.5)	+ 9.3 (17.2)	+ 6.4 (17.4)	NS	NS
Full Scale IQ (Prorated)	+ 5.3 (21.9)	- 0.1 (26.0)	+ 8.1 (20.9)	+ 6.9 (16.9)	+ 4.9 (15.8)	NS	NS
EH-3 Reading Quotient	+ 2.8 (15.3)	- 0.2 (16.5)	+ 4.8 (17.6)	- 3.4 (14.8)	+ 4.6 (13.2)	NS	NS

Table 36 (Continued)

MEAN CASE-CONTROL DIFFERENCES IN PSYCHOLOGICAL TEST SCORES AND FREQUENCY OF SOLVENT ABUSE IN PAIRS MATCHED FOR ETHNIC BACKGROUND

	Frequency of Solvent Abuse						
	1-2 Times	3-4 Times	5-9 Times	10-30 Times	>30 Times		Test for linear trend
	(N=27)	(N=11)	(N=11)	(N=15)	(N=14)	Sig	Sig
Passage Recall: Items Recalled							
Immediate Presentation	+ 0.3 (5.2)	+ 2.0 (6.7)	+ 0.5 (5.0)	+ 1.2 (6.3)	+ 0.9 (3.8)	NS	NS
Delayed Presentation	+ 0.7 (5.2)	+ 1.8 (6.1)	+ 0.8 (4.6)	+ 0.8 (6.1)	+ 1.6 (3.7)	NS	NS
Speed of Information Processing							
T-Score	+ 2.0 (10.5)	+ 1.1 (10.4)	+ 1.6 (10.0)	- 0.4 (8.5)	+ 3.1 (11.4)	NS	NS
Manual Dexterity							
Right hand (Time in secs)	+ 0.0 (1.6)	- 1.0 (1.6)	+ 0.2 (1.1)	+ 0.1 (1.0)	+ 0.2 (1.5)	NS	NS
Left hand (Time in secs)	+ 0.1 (1.7)	- 0.8 (2.0)	+ 0.1 (1.9)	+ 0.3 (0.9)	+ 0.0 (1.5)	NS	NS
Vibration Perception Threshold							
Thumb	- 0.0 (1.9)	- 0.2 (1.2)	- 0.1 (1.3)	- 0.6 (1.1)	- 0.4 (4.0)	NS	NS
Ankle	- 0.7 (3.3)	- 1.0 (2.3)	+ 0.3 (2.0)	+ 0.1 (2.0)	+ 2.6 (10.2)	NS	*

* $p < 0.05$

Table 36 (Continued)

MEAN CASE-CONTROL DIFFERENCE IN PSYCHOLOGICAL TEST SCORES AND FREQUENCY OF SOLVENT ABUSE IN PAIRS MATCHED FOR ETHNIC BACKGROUND

	Frequency of Solvent Abuse						
	1-2 Times	3-4 Times	5-9 Times	10-30 Times	> 30 Times		Test for linear trend
	(N=27)	(N=11)	(N=11)	(N=15)	(N=14)	Sig	Sig
Bexley-Maudsley Automated Tests							
Visual Discrimination							
Mean RT: Grade 2	- 0.22 (1.82)	- 0.38 (2.02)	+ 0.33 (1.47)	- 1.49 (2.54)	- 0.07 (1.46)	NS	NS
Mean RT: Grade 4	- 0.26 (1.27)	- 0.15 (1.51)	- 0.39 (1.27)	- 0.08 (1.94)	- 0.05 (1.66)	NS	NS
Errors: Grade 2	- 0.4 (2.0)	+ 0.0 (1.7)	- 0.2 (2.4)	- 0.4 (0.9)	- 0.2 (2.0)	NS	NS
Errors: Grade 4	- 0.3 (1.4)	- 0.4 (0.8)	+ 0.2 (1.1)	- 0.1 (0.8)	+ 0.6 (1.7)	NS	*
Symbol-digit Coding							
Mean RT: 1st 15	- 0.03 (0.31)	- 0.04 (0.27)	- 0.16 (0.29)	- 0.12 (0.67)	- 0.19 (0.30)	NS	NS
Mean RT: 2nd 15	- 0.02 (0.25)	- 0.12 (0.33)	- 0.07 (0.33)	- 0.12 (0.58)	- 0.14 (0.47)	NS	NS
Mean RT: 3rd 15	+ 0.05 (0.30)	- 0.01 (0.36)	+ 0.01 (0.23)	- 0.14 (0.63)	- 0.16 (0.25)	NS	NS
Mean RT: All 45	+ 0.00 (0.22)	- 0.06 (0.26)	- 0.08 (0.20)	- 0.13 (0.57)	- 0.16 (0.29)	NS	NS
Mistakes: All 45	+ 0.8 (2.6)	+ 0.2 (1.2)	- 1.1 (1.9)	- 0.7 (2.4)	- 0.4 (1.4)	NS	NS

* $p < 0.05$

Table 36 (continued)

MEAN CASE-CONTROL DIFFERENCE IN PSYCHOLOGICAL TEST SCORES AND FREQUENCY OF SOLVENT ABUSE IN PAIRS MATCHED FOR ETHNIC BACKGROUND

	Frequency of Solvent Abuse						
	1-2 Times	3-4 Times	5-9 Times	10-30 Times	> 30 Times		Test for linear trend
	(N=27)	(N=11)	(N=11)	(N=15)	(N=14)	Sig	Sig
Reaction Time Tests							
A) Two choice Mean RT:							
Either Hand	-0.043 (0.088)	+0.031 (0.081)	+0.021 (0.070)	-0.037 (0.136)	+0.012 (0.058)	NS	NS
Left-Right Errors	+0.4 (1.5)	+0.0 (1.7)	-0.4 (1.6)	+0.6 (1.8)	+0.0 (0.9)	NS	NS
B) Two choice with Inhibition Mean RT:							
Either Hand	-0.077 (0.174)	-0.007 (0.158)	-0.008 (0.180)	-0.011 (0.207)	-0.027 (0.126)	NS	NS
Failed Inhibitory Response	-0.4 (1.7)	-0.6 (0.8)	-1.4 (2.9)	-1.6 (2.9)	+0.9 (2.9)	NS	NS
Finger Tapping (Taps per sec)							
Right Hand Index	+0.3 (2.1)	-0.5 (1.1)	-1.7 (2.0)	-0.5 (2.2)	-0.2 (1.9)	NS	NS
Left Hand Index	+0.6 (1.7)	+0.8 (2.3)	-0.7 (1.0)	+0.3 (1.8)	-0.7 (1.3)	NS	NS
Right Hand Index/Middle	+0.2 (1.0)	-0.1 (1.1)	-0.5 (1.0)	-0.2 (0.8)	-0.4 (1.3)	NS	NS
Left Hand Index/Middle	+0.1 (1.1)	-0.3 (0.8)	-0.3 (1.0)	+0.0 (1.3)	-1.0 (1.0)	NS	NS
Right/Left Hand Index	-0.0 (1.1)	-0.6 (0.9)	-0.6 (0.6)	-0.5 (2.5)	-1.1 (0.7)	NS	NS
Trial Making (Secs per target)							
1-9 (Not Practice Item)	+0.5 (1.0)	-0.2 (0.5)	+0.4 (1.1)	-0.4 (0.8)	-0.1 (0.9)	NS	NS
1-9 Alternating	+0.1 (1.1)	-0.9 (1.3)	+0.9 (0.9)	-0.1 (0.9)	+0.0 (1.0)	NS	NS

Table 37

SUMMARY OF STATISTICALLY SIGNIFICANT RELATIONSHIPS BETWEEN SOLVENT ABUSE AND PSYCHOLOGICAL TEST VARIABLES (ANALYSES OF CONTROL-MINUS-CASE DIFFERENCES) IN PAIRS MATCHED FOR ETHNIC BACKGROUND

	Case V Control	Freq. of solvent abuse	Time since last abused solvents	Number of different products abused	Time since first abused solvents
WISC					
Similarities	-	-	-	-	-
Vocabulary	*	-	-	-	-
Picture Completion	-	-	-	-	-
Block design	-	-	*	-	-
Verbal IQ	*	-	-	-	-
Performance IQ	-	-	*	-	-
Full Scale IQ	*	-	-	-	-
EH-3 READING QUOTIENT	-	-	-	-	-
PASSAGE RECALL					
Immediate presentation	-	-	-	-	-
Delayed presentation	-	-	-	-	-
SPEED OF INFORMATION PROCESSING	-	-	-	-	-
MANUAL DEXTERITY					
Right hand	-	-	-	-	-
Left hand	-	-	-	-	-
VIBRATION SENSATION THRESHOLD					
Thumb	-	-	-	-	-
Ankle	-	-	-	*	-
BMAPS: VISUAL DISCRIMINATION					
Mean RT: grade 2	-	-	-	-	-
Mean RT: grade 4	-	-	-	-	-
Errors: grade 2	-	-	-	-	-
Errors: grade 4	-	-	-	-	*
BMAPS: SYMBOL-DIGIT CODING					
Mean RT: 1st 15	-	-	-	-	-
Mean RT: 2nd 15	-	-	-	-	-
Mean RT: 3rd 15	-	-	-	-	-
Mean RT: all 45	-	-	-	-	-
Mistakes: all 45	-	-	-	-	-
RT: 2 CHOICE					
Mean RT: either hand	-	-	-	-	*
Left-right errors	-	-	*	-	-
RT: 2 CHOICE WITH INHIBITION					
Mean RT: either hand	-	-	-	-	-
Failed inhibitory responses	*	-	-	-	-
FINGER TAPPING					
Right hand index	-	-	*	-	*
Left hand index	-	-	-	-	-
Right hand index/middle	-	-	-	-	*
Left hand index/middle	-	-	-	-	-
Right/left hand index	-	-	-	-	-
TRAIL-MAKING TASK					
1-9	-	-	-	-	-
1-9 alternating	-	-	-	-	-

* $p < 0.05$

Table 38

TESTS FROM WHICH VALID DATA ON ANTECEDENTS EDUCATIONAL ATTAINMENT WERE OBTAINED

	Cases (n=105)	Controls (n=105)
Reading Tests		
London Reading Test	18	18
Neale Analysis of Reading Ability	14	17
Schonell Graded Word Reading Test	4	4
Holborn Reading Test	1	1
Burt Word Reading Test	1	0
Verbal Reasoning Tests		
NFER	22	26
Cognitive Abilities Test (Verbal Quotient)	11	13
Moray House Verbal Reasoning Test 91	2	3
	73 (69.5%)	83 (79.0%)

Table 39

ANTECEDENT AND CURRENT (INITIAL ASSESSMENT) TEST SCORES IN PAIRS MATCHED FOR ETHNIC BACKGROUND

	Antecedent test scores	Current test scores	Change over time
A) Reading Ability			
Controls (N=19)	103.5 (11.2)	106.6 (15.2)	+ 3.1
			NS
Solvent Abusers (N = 19)	103.1 (13.0)	100.3 (13.0)	- 2.8
B) Verbal Reasoning or Verbal IQ			
Controls (N = 21)	104.3 (12.4)	107.6 (16.2)	+ 3.3
			*
Solvent Abusers (N = 21)	110.6 (10.9)	105.6 (17.0)	- 5.0

* $p < 0.05$

Table 40

AGE, SCHOOL YEAR, SEX AND ETHNIC BACKGROUND (FOLLOW-UP)

	Controls (N=71)		Solvent abusers (N=61)	
Age				
In Months (Mean and S.D.)	186.3	(7.5)	185.9	(6.2)
In Years				
14	16	(22.5%)	10	(16.4%)
15	36	(50.7%)	40	(65.6%)
16	19	(26.8%)	11	(18.0%)
School Year				
4th Year	20	(28.2%)	17	(27.9%)
5th Year	51	(71.8%)	44	(72.1%)
Sex				
Boys	29	(40.8%)	23	(37.7%)
Girls	42	(59.1%)	38	(62.3%)
Ethnic Background				*
White	53	(74.6%)	55	(90.2%)
Afro-Caribbean	15	(21.1%)	4	(6.6%)
Indian Subcontinent	3	(4.2%)	2	(3.3%)

* $p < 0.05$

Table 41

ILLNESSES AND ACCIDENTS BETWEEN INITIAL AND FOLLOW-UP ASSESSMENT

	Controls (N=71)	Solvent abusers (N=61)	Signif
Since Initial Assessment			
Missed school at all because of illness	41 (57.7%)	36 (59.0%)	NS
Off school for a week or more because of illness	19 (26.8%)	16 (26.2%)	NS
Took prescribed medicines	8 (11.3%)	6 (9.8%)	NS
Hospital treatment or admission for accident or illness	8 (11.3%)	17 (27.9%)	*

* $p < 0.05$

Table 42

FREQUENCY OF SOLVENT ABUSE BY CASES AND CONTROLS
BETWEEN INITIAL AND FOLLOW-UP ASSESSMENTS

Frequency of	Controls		Cases	
solvent abuse	n	%	n	%
Not at all	71	(98.6)	46	(75.4)
1 - 2 Times	1*	(1.4)	4	(6.6)
3 - 4 Times	0		4	(6.6)
5 - 9 Times	0		4	(6.6)
10 - 30 Times	0		3	(4.9)
> 30 Times	0		0	(0.0)
Total	72	(100.0)	61	(100.0)

*Excluded from follow-up assessment

Table 43

MOST RECENT EPISODE OF SOLVENT ABUSE BY CASES ASSESSED AT FOLLOW-UP

	Cases	
	n	%
Yesterday	0	0.0
2-3 days ago	0	0.0
4-7 days ago	2	3.5
1 week - 1 month	3	5.3
1-3 months	6	10.5
3-6 months	2	3.5
6-12 months	9	15.8
> 12 months	35	57.4
Not Known	4	
TOTAL	61	100.0

Table 44

ILLICIT DRUG USE (EVER) BY CASES AND CONTROLS ASSESSED AT FOLLOW-UP

	Controls		Solvent abusers		
	(N=71)		(N=61)		P
Cannabis	9	(12.7%)	48	(78.7%)	***
Amphetamines	0	(0.0%)	13	(21.3%)	***
Cocaine or heroin	0	(0.0%)	3	(4.9%)	NS
LSD	0	(0.0%)	2	(3.2%)	NS
Other	0	(0.0%)	2	(3.2%)	NS

*** $p < 0.001$

Table 45

PSYCHOLOGICAL TEST SCORES OF CASES AND CONTROLS
MATCHED FOR ETHNIC BACKGROUND AT FOLLOW-UP
(READMINISTERED TESTS)

	Controls (N=38)	Solvent abusers (N=38)	Signif
WISC			
Similarities	12.0 (2.6)	11.1 (2.8)	NS
Vocabulary	10.0 (2.3)	9.4 (2.4)	NS
Picture Completion	12.3 (2.6)	12.7 (2.6)	NS
Block Design	12.5 (2.6)	12.5 (2.4)	NS
Verbal IQ (prorated)	106.2 (12.9)	101.6 (14.6)	NS
Performance IQ (prorated)	117.1 (14.4)	118.3 (14.7)	NS
Full Scale IQ (prorated)	112.5 (11.8)	110.4 (13.8)	NS
EH-3 Reading Quotient	Not readministered		

144

Table 45 (continued)

PSYCHOLOGICAL TEST SCORES OF CASES AND CONTROLS
MATCHED FOR ETHNIC BACKGROUND AT FOLLOW-UP
(READMINISTERED TESTS)

	Controls (N=38)	Solvent abusers (N=38)	Signif
Passage Recall: Items Recalled			
Immediate Presentation	9.7 (2.9)	8.6 (3.2)	NS
Delayed Presentation	8.8 (2.6)	7.5 (3.1)	NS
Speed of Information Processing			
T-Score	Not readministered		
Manual Dexterity			
Right Hand (Time in Secs)	9.6 (0.7)	9.8 (1.1)	NS
Left Hand (Time in Secs)	10.3 (0.8)	10.4 (1.4)	NS
Vibration Sensation Threshold	Not readministered		

Table 46

PSYCHOLOGICAL TEST SCORES OF CASES AND CONTROLS
MATCHED FOR ETHNIC BACKGROUND AT FOLLOW-UP
(NEWLY -INTRODUCED TESTS)

	Controls (N=38)	Solvent abusers (N=38)	Sig
British Picture Vocabulary Test			
Standardized Score	96.5 (13.4)	93.9 (11.6)	NS
Gibson Spiral Maze			
Mean Time Taken (in secs)	37.8 (11.2)	38.6 (10.0)	NS
Errors	7.9 (5.6)	8.7 (6.5)	NS
Matching Familiar Figures			
Mean Latency (in secs)	9.5 (3.7)	10.4 (4.9)	NS
Total Errors	4.0 (2.2)	4.9 (2.8)	NS
Items Correct First Trial	6.4 (1.7)	6.1 (2.0)	NS
Extended Symbol Digit Coding Test			
Mean RT: All 225	1.55 (0.29)	1.61 (0.31)	NS
Mistakes: All 225	18.3 (23.4)	19.5 (25.4)	NS
Items Recalled (out of 10)	6.8 (2.1)	6.7 (2.1)	NS
Mean RT: 1st 45	1.68 (0.25)	1.75 (0.29)	NS

Table 46 (continued)

PSYCHOLOGICAL TEST SCORES OF CASES AND CONTROLS MATCHED FOR ETHNIC BACKGROUND AT FOLLOW-UP (NEWLY INTRODUCED TESTS)

	Controls (N=38)	Solvent abusers (N=38)	Signif
Extended Symbol-digit Coding Test			
Mean RT: 1st 15	1.74 (0.28)	1.84 (0.30)	NS
Mean RT: 2nd 15	1.69 (0.26)	1.71 (0.34)	NS
Mean RT: 3rd 15	1.62 (0.27)	1.70 (0.31)	NS
Mean RT: 4th 15	1.62 (0.44)	1.66 (0.29)	NS
Mean RT: 5th 15	1.50 (0.41)	1.67 (0.38)	NS
Mean RT: 6th 15	1.64 (0.35)	1.68 (0.32)	NS
Mean RT: 7th 15	1.64 (0.45)	1.68 (0.41)	NS
Mean RT: 8th 15	1.48 (0.31)	1.61 (0.52)	NS
Mean RT: 9th 15	1.53 (0.30)	1.59 (0.38)	NS
Mean RT: 10th 15	1.58 (0.43)	1.56 (0.39)	NS
Mean RT: 11th 15	1.44 (0.30)	1.49 (0.39)	NS
Mean RT: 12th 15	1.49 (0.28)	1.57 (0.37)	NS
Mean RT: 13th 15	1.32 (0.27)	1.40 (0.39)	NS
Mean RT: 14th 15	1.46 (0.28)	1.72 (1.00)	NS
Mean RT: 15th 15	1.38 (0.29)	1.44 (0.40)	NS

Table 47

PREVALENCE SURVEYS OF SOLVENT ABUSE

Survey	Place	Year Done	Age Range	N. of Schools	N. of Children	Substance(s) Asked About	Positive Respondents
British							
Ramsey (1982)	Glasgow	1976	11-16	1	898	Solvents	9.8%
Plant et al (1984/5)	Edinburgh	1979	15-16	5	1036	Glues & solvents	4.6%
NOP Ltd (1982)	G.B.	1982	15-21	*	1326	Glue	3.0%
Lynch (1984)	Berkshire	NK	?	7	?	Solvents	8.5%
Stuart (1986)	Macclesfield	1985	11-18	*	1729	Solvents	6.0%
Williams (1986)	UK	NK	>14<19	*	2417	Solvents	6.0%
Faber (1985)	East Sussex	1983	11-18	9	7343	Solvents	8.1%
Pritchard et al (1986)	Bournemouth & Soton	1985	14-16	6	808	Solvents	12.4%
Diamond et al (1988)	Bournemouth & Soton	1986	14-16		602	Solvents	8.8%
Cooke et al (1988)	South Wales	1985	11-18	+28	4474	Solvents	6.8%
Swadi (1988)	London	NK	11-16	6	3073	Solvents	11.0%
Canada							
Whitehead (1970)	Halifax	1969	12-19	*	1606	Glue (in past 6 mo)	3.1%
Fejer et al (1972)	Halifax, Canada	1970	12-19	*	1081	Glue (in past 6 mo)	7.2%
Smart & Fejer (1975)	Toronto, Canada	1968	12-19	*	6447	Glue (in past 6 mo)	5.7%
		1970	12-19	*	6890	Glue (in past 6 mo)	3.8%
		1972	12-19	*	?	Glue (in past 6 mo)	2.9%
		1974	12-19	*	?	Glue (in past 6 mo)	3.8%

Reference	Location	Year	Age		n	Substance	%
Smart et al (1985)	Ontario, Canada	1977	12-19*		4687	Glue (in past year)	3.9%
						Other (in past year)	6.6%
		1979	12-19	*	4794	Glue (in past year)	3.9%
						Other (in past year)	6.2%
		1981	12-19	*	3270	Glue (in past year)	2.3%
						Other (in past year)	3.2%
		1983	12-19	*	4737	Glue (in past year)	3.2%
		1985	12-19	*	4154	Glue (in past year)	2.0%
						Other (in past year)	2.7%
USA							
Fishburne et al (1980)	USA	1979	12-17	*	2165	Inhalants	9.8%
Johnston et al (1984)	USA	1983	Seniors	*	app 16000	Inhalants + nitrites	18.8%
Johnson et al (1971)	Oregon	1968	Fr-Sens	18	2777	Inhalants approx	15.0%
Gossett et al (1971)	Dallas, Texas	1969	12-18	43	56745	Airplane glue	10.1%
Porter et al (1973)	Anchorage, Alaska	1971	10-20	51	15634	Solvents	16.6%
Kandel et al (1976)	New York State	1971	Fr-Sens	18	8206	Inhalants	8.0%
Yancy et al (1972)	Monroe Co. NY	1971	15-18	28	7228	Glue	7.2%
Stephens et al (1978)	New York State	1974/5	>11 >18	*	8553	Solvents	5.2%
Schaffer (1984)	Mobile, Alabama	1981	12-?	?	app 25000	Glue, aerosols etc	7.6%
Mexican							
Castro et al (1980)	Mexico City	1978/9	>14 >18	*	4059	Inhalants	5.4%
Australian							
Dunoon & Hornel (1984)	New South Wales	1983	12-17	29	4165	Solvents	54.1%
Min. Educ. (1986)	Victoria	NK	12-17	*	2538	Inhalants approx	27.0%

* Stratified sampling within schools
Fr-Sens: Freshmen & Seniors

Figure 1

DERIVATION OF THE CASE AND CONTROL GROUPS FOR DETAILED ASSESSMENT

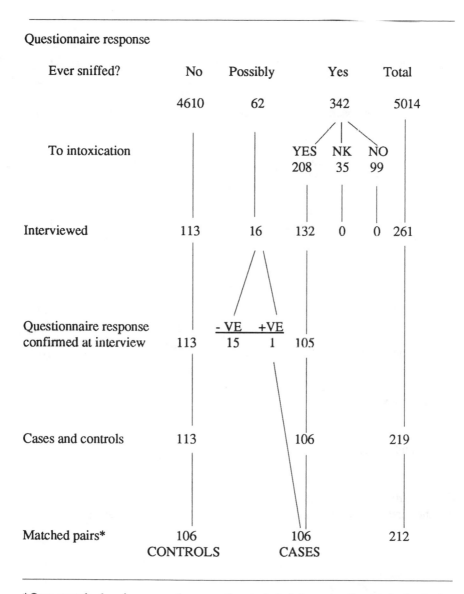

Questionnaire response

Ever sniffed?	No	Possibly		Yes		Total
	4610	62		342		5014

To intoxication — YES 208, NK 35, NO 99

Interviewed — 113, 16, 132, 0, 0, 261

Questionnaire response confirmed at interview — 113, -VE 15, +VE 1, 105

Cases and controls — 113, 106, 219

Matched pairs* — 106 CONTROLS, 106 CASES, 212

*One matched pair was subsequently excluded because the toxicological examination of the control was positive.

Figure 2
THE FOLLOW-UP SAMPLES

Group	Solvent abusers				Controls			
Initial school year	**3rd**	**4th**	**5th**	**Total**	**3rd**	**4th**	**5th**	**Total**
Initial assessment samples	20	61	24	105	20	61	24	105
No attempt to trace: initially tested in 1983/4 or 1985/6		3				4		
Attempted to trace: initially tested in 1984/5	20	58		78	20	57		77
Attending another school or Support Unit		4				1		
Still at same school	20	54		73	19	57		76
Absent from school	2	11				4		
Found and tested	18 +	43	=	61	19 +	53	=	72

One control was subsequently excluded because she had abused solvents for the first time during the interval between the two assessments.

LOKI: AGENT OF ASGARD VOL. 2 — I CANNOT TELL A LIE. Contains material originally published in magazine form as LOKI: AGENT OF ASGARD #6-11. First printing 2015. ISBN# 978-0-7851-9331-9. Published by MARVEL WORLDWIDE, INC., a subsidiary of MARVEL ENTERTAINMENT, LLC. OFFICE OF PUBLICATION: 135 West 50th Street, New York, NY 10020. Copyright © 2015 MARVEL. No similarity between any of the names, characters, persons, and/or institutions in this magazine with those of any living or dead person or institution is intended, and any such similarity which may exist is purely coincidental. Printed in Canada. ALAN FINE, President, Marvel Entertainment; DAN BUCKLEY, President, TV, Publishing and Brand Management; JOE QUESADA, Chief Creative Officer; TOM BREVOORT, SVP of Publishing; DAVID BOGART, SVP of Operations & Procurement, Publishing; C.B. CEBULSKI, SVP of Creator & Content Development; DAVID GABRIEL, SVP Print, Sales & Marketing; JIM O'KEEFE, VP of Operations & Logistics; DAN CARR, Executive Director of Publishing Technology; SUSAN CRESPI, Editorial Operations Manager; ALEX MORALES, Publishing Operations Manager; STAN LEE, Chairman Emeritus. For information regarding advertising in Marvel Comics or on Marvel.com, please contact Niza Disla, Director of Marvel Partnerships, at ndisla@marvel.com. For Marvel subscription inquiries, please call 800-217-9158. Manufactured between 2/27/2015 and 4/6/2015 by SOLISCO PRINTERS, SCOTT, QC, CANADA.

10 9 8 7 6 5 4 3 2 1

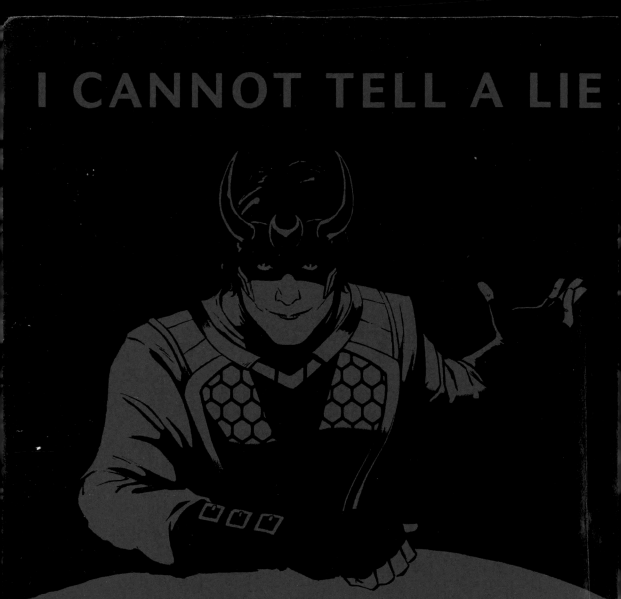

I CANNOT TELL A LIE

WRITER	**AL EWING**
ARTISTS	**JORGE COELHO** (#6-7) &
	LEE GARBETT (#8-11)
COLOR ARTISTS	**LEE LOUGHRIDGE** (#6-7),
	NOLAN WOODARD (#8-10) &
	ANTONIO FABELA (#11)
LETTERER	**VC's CLAYTON COWLES**
COVER ARTIST	**LEE GARBETT**
ASSISTANT EDITOR	**JON MOISAN**
EDITOR	**WIL MOSS**

LOKI CREATED BY STAN LEE, LARRY LIEBER & JACK KIRBY

Collection Editor: Jennifer Grönwald · Assistant Editor: Sarah Brunstad · Associate Managing Editor: Alex Starbuck
Editor, Special Projects: Mark D. Beazley · Senior Editor, Special Projects: Jeff Youngquist · SVP Print, Sales & Marketing: David Gabriel

Editor in Chief: Axel Alonso · Chief Creative Officer: Joe Quesada · Publisher: Dan Buckley · Executive Producer: Alan Fine

THIS IS THE STORY OF LOKI.

LOKI, WHO WORKED FOR THE ALL-MOTHER AS THEIR AGENT, ERASING ONE CRIME FROM HIS PAST FOR EVERY MISSION HE COMPLETED. WHO HOPED, IN THIS WAY, TO ESCAPE HIS OLD STORY. WHO HOPED TO CHANGE.

LOKI, WHO WITH HIS FRIENDS — HIS BROTHER THOR, THE ASGARDIAN LORELEI AND VERITY WILLIS, A HUMAN WITH THE POWER TO SEE THROUGH ANY LIE — BROKE INTO THE DUNGEONS OF ASGARDIA TO LEARN THE SECRET TRUTH THAT LAY BEHIND HIS MISSIONS.

AND THERE FOUND A SECOND LOKI — AN OLD LOKI. THE AGENT OF AN OLDER ASGARD, ABLE TO WALK FREELY IN TIME, WHO HAS RETURNED TO THE PRESENT FROM THE END OF ALL THINGS TO ENSURE HIS FUTURE COMES TO BE. A GOLDEN FUTURE OF PEACE AND PLENTY THAT THE ALL-MOTHER ALSO WISHES TO SEE COME TO PASS — BUT A FUTURE IN WHICH LOKI WILL NOT AND CANNOT CHANGE HIS STORY. A FUTURE THAT TRAPS HIM FOREVER — WITH THE ALL-MOTHER'S KNOWLEDGE AND CONSENT.

LOKI, BETRAYED, QUIT THE ALL-MOTHER'S SERVICE, AND AIDED HIS BROTHER THOR IN SEEKING THE TRUTH ABOUT THEIR HERETOFORE-UNKNOWN SISTER — ANGELA, GUARDIAN OF THE GALAXY, RAISED IN THE TENTH REALM OF HEVEN BY THE ASGARD-HATING ANGELIC HOST. IN THE PROCESS, LOKI RETRIEVED ODIN FROM HIS LONG EXILE IN THE REMAINS OF ASGARD-SPACE AND RETURNED HIM TO ASGARDIA. IT WAS A RICH, FULL DAY, AND IT TOOK HIS MIND OFF THINGS.

(IT WAS A FULL DAY FOR THE OLDER LOKI, TOO, WHO MEDDLED IN THE EVENTS FROM AFAR — ONLY TO FIND HIS DESIRE FOR CHAOS THWARTED.)

BUT NOW THE YOUNG LOKI HAS RETURNED TO HIS APARTMENT IN MANHATTAN AND HIS LIFE AMONG THE MORTALS, WITH NO IDEA WHAT HIS NEXT MOVE WILL BE...BUT WITH A COLD CERTAINTY THAT SOMEWHERE, IN A DANK CELL IN ASGARDIA OR AT THE END OF TIME, THERE LURKS HIS EVIL FUTURE SELF...

...THE AGENT OF ASGARD.

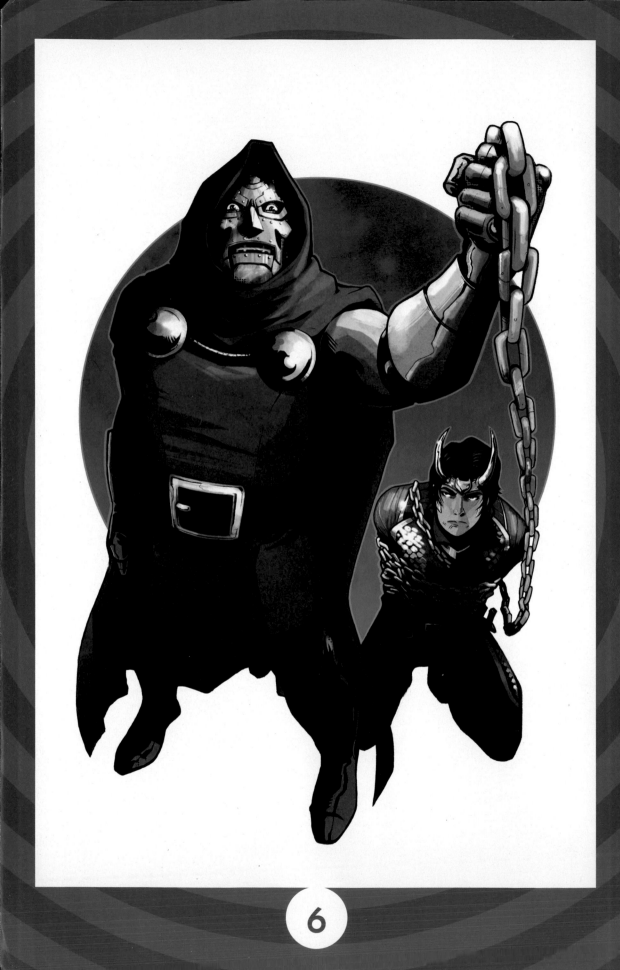

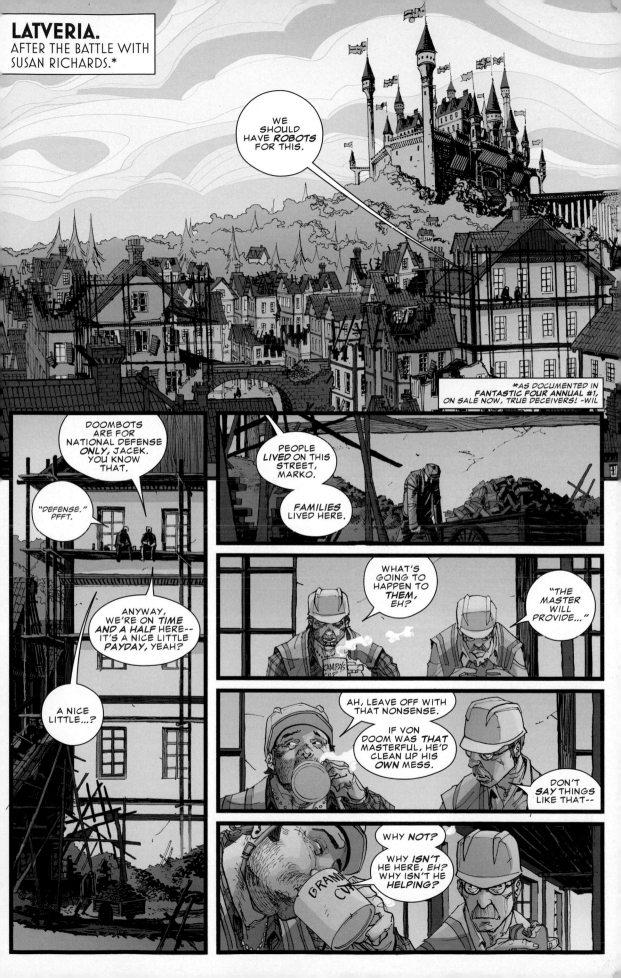

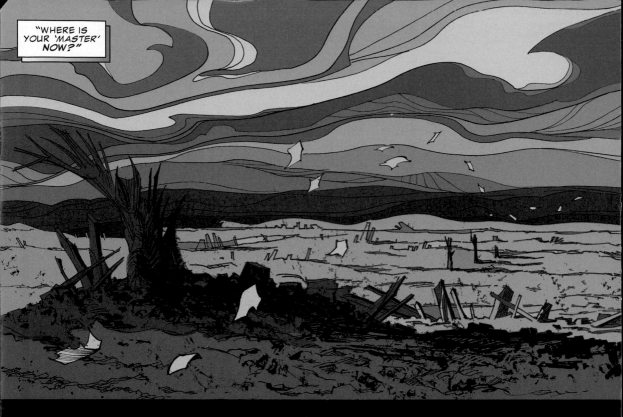

"WHERE IS YOUR 'MASTER' NOW?"

DEGREE

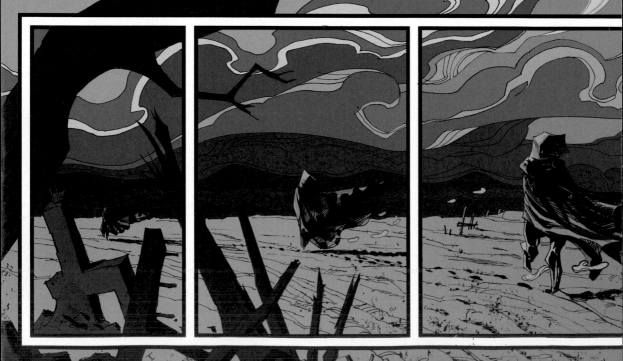

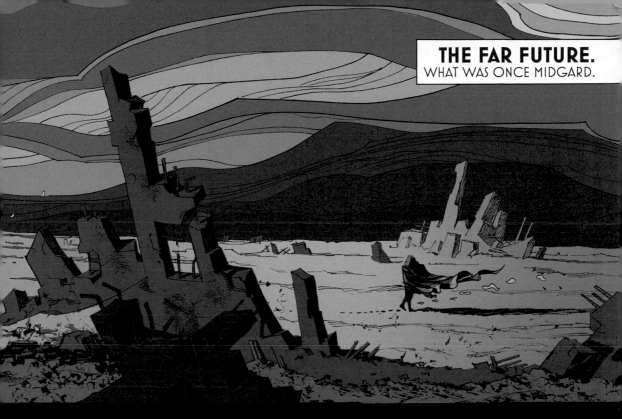

THE FAR FUTURE.
WHAT WAS ONCE MIDGARD.

ABSOLUTE

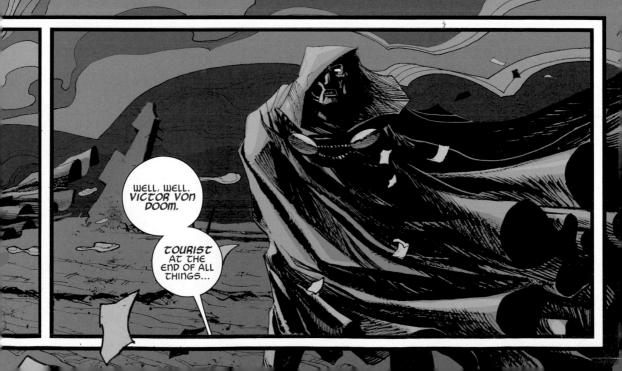

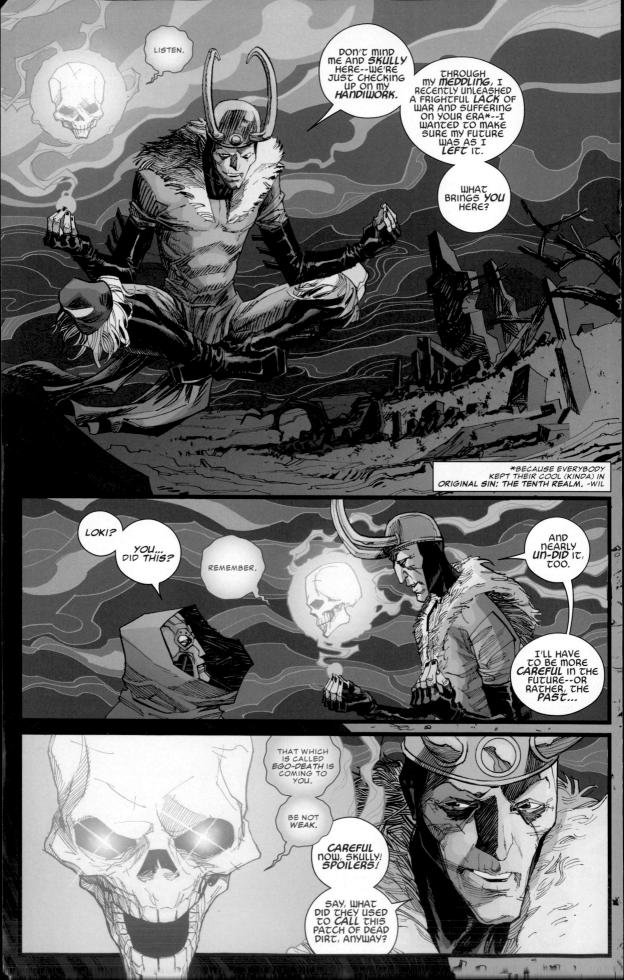

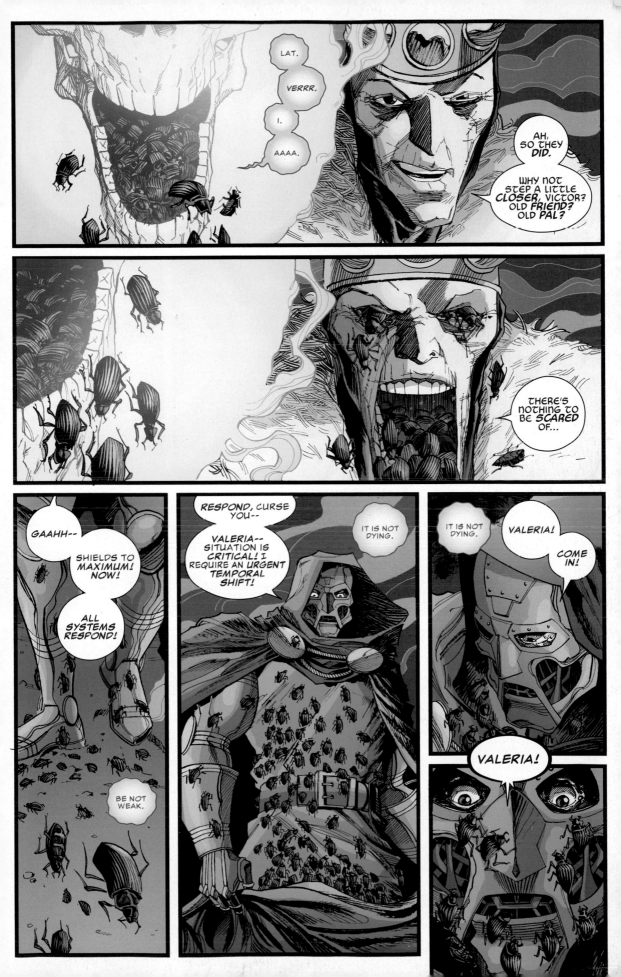

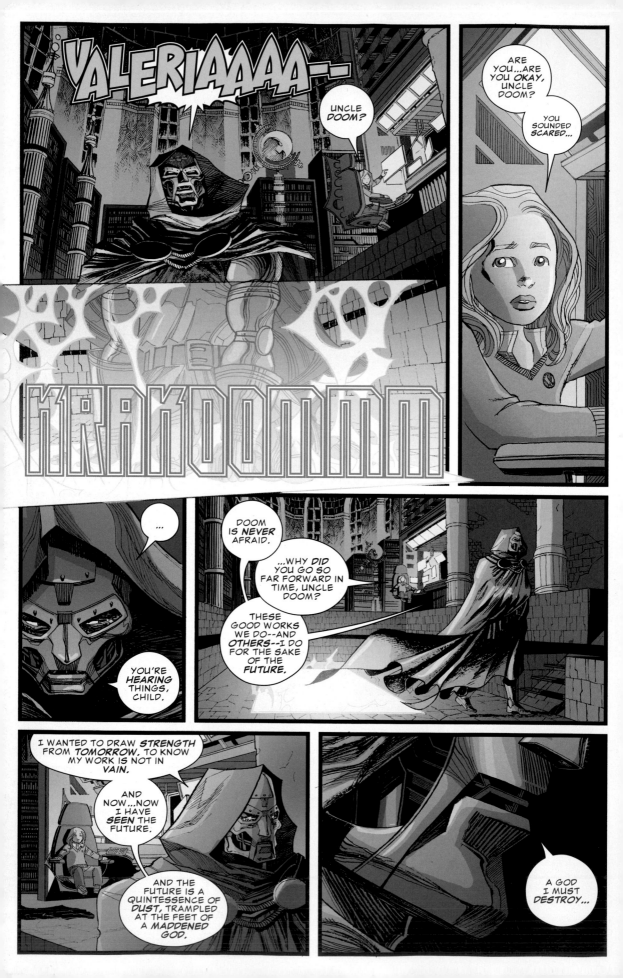

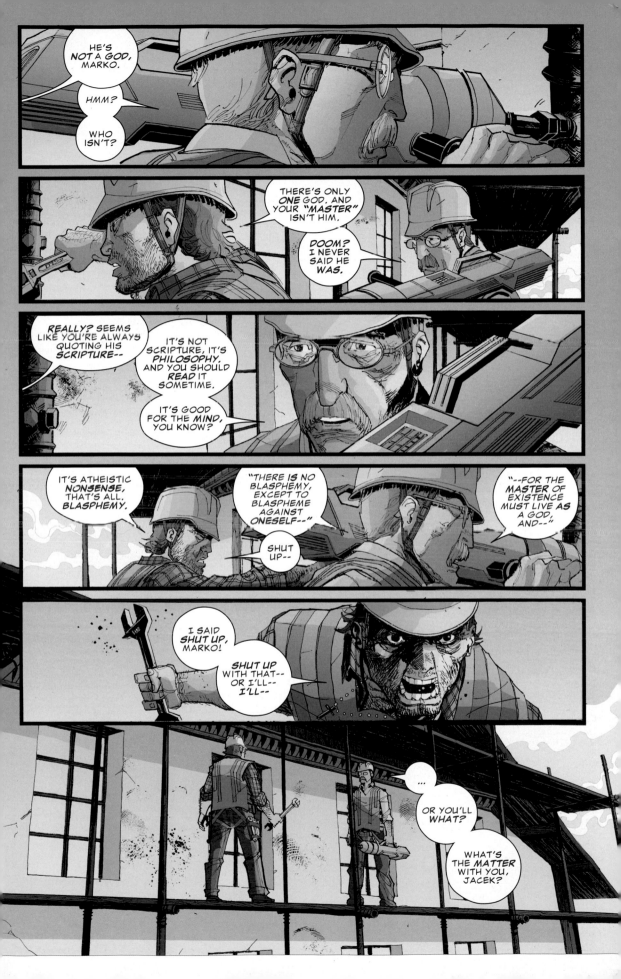

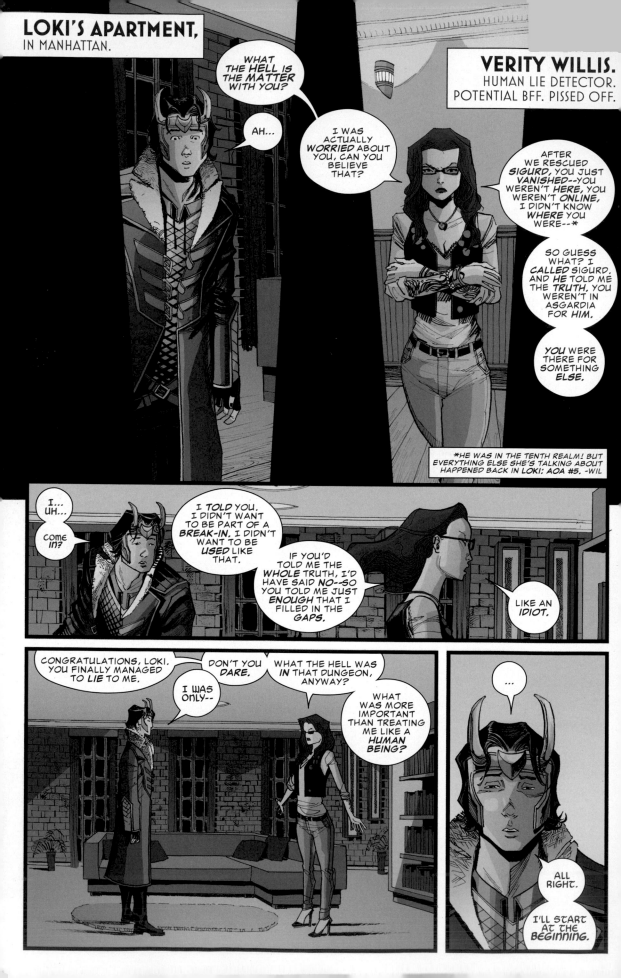

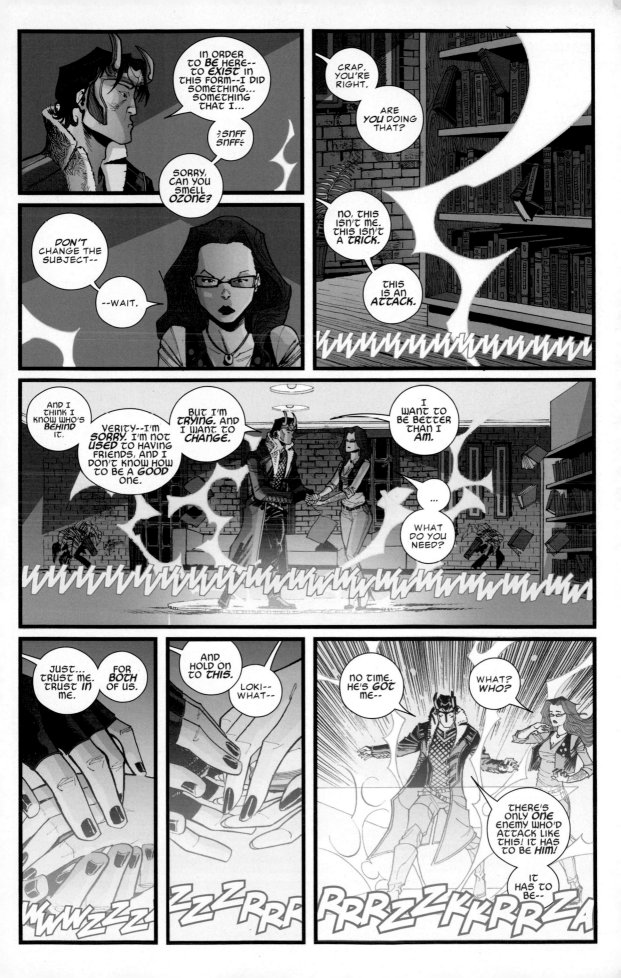

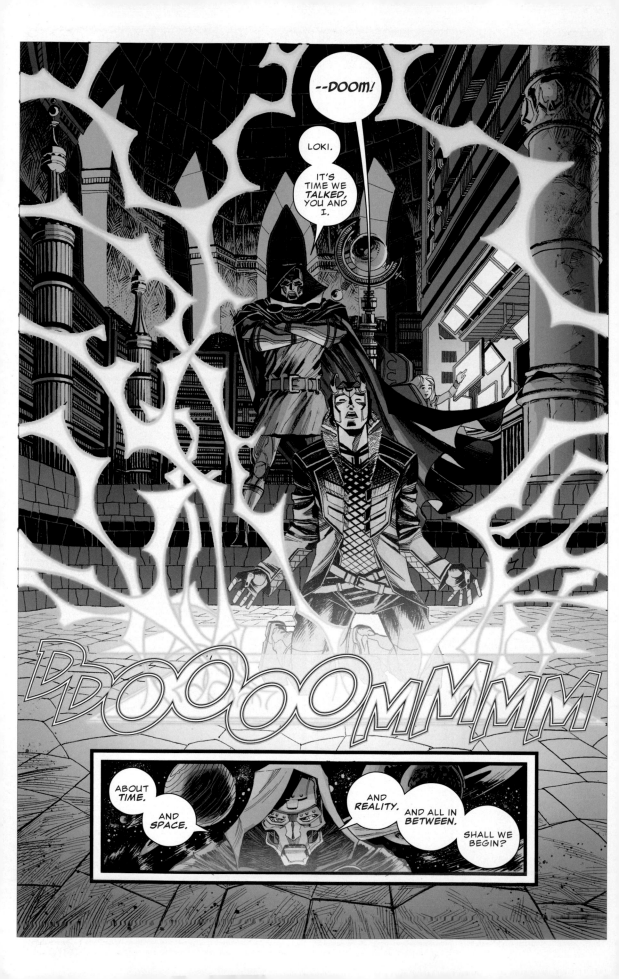

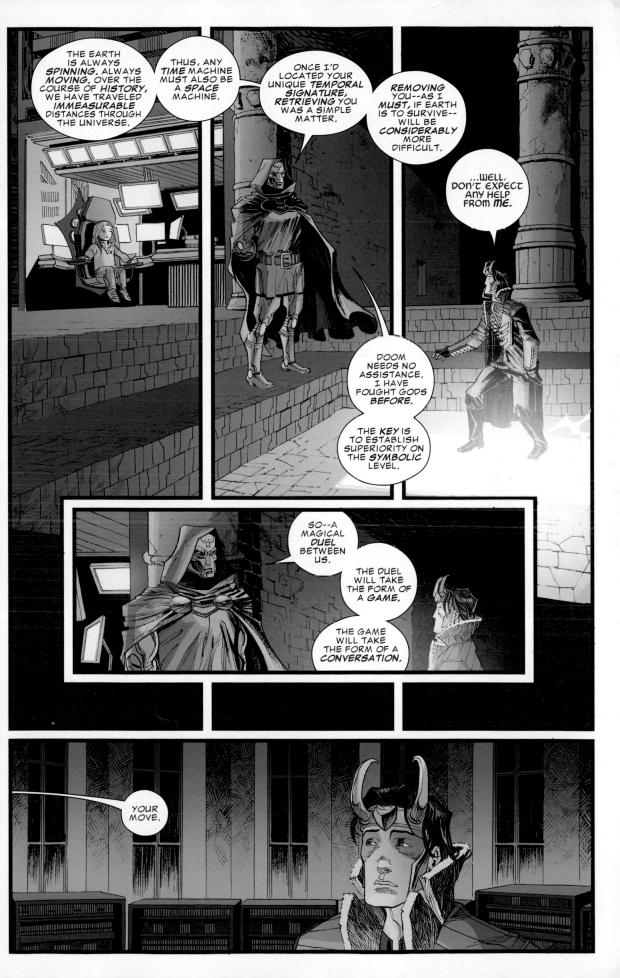

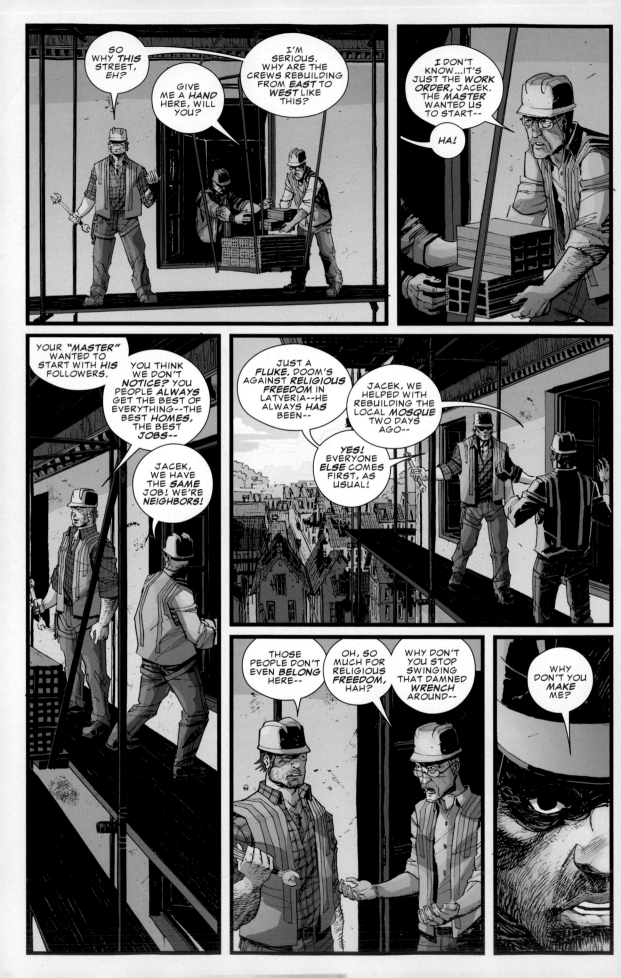

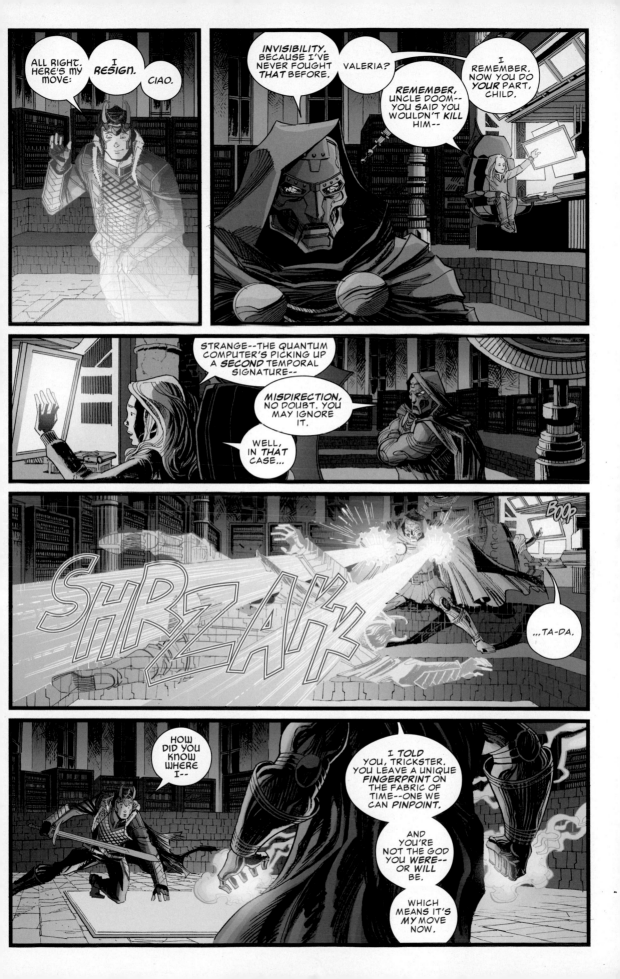

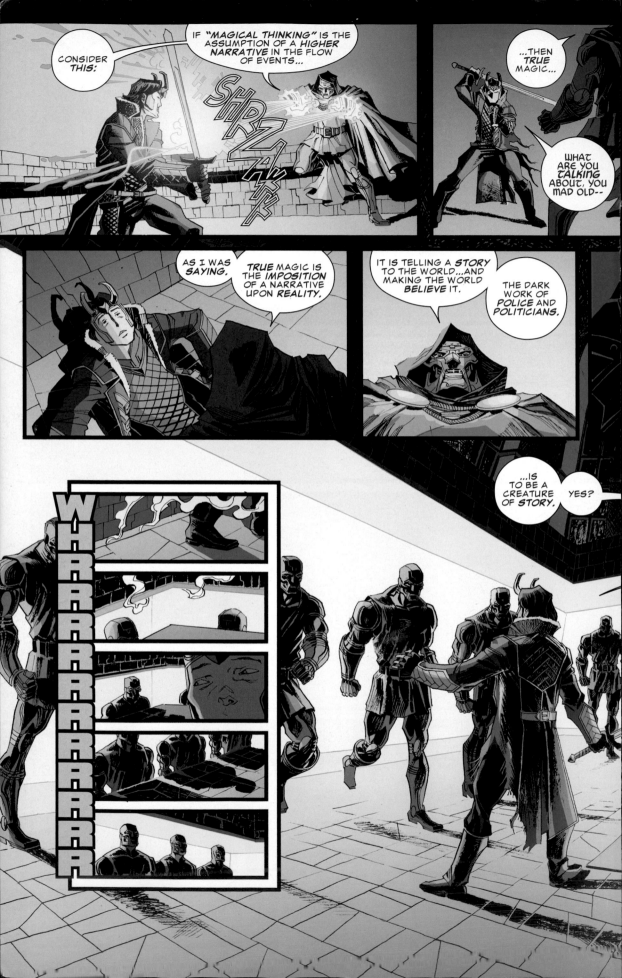

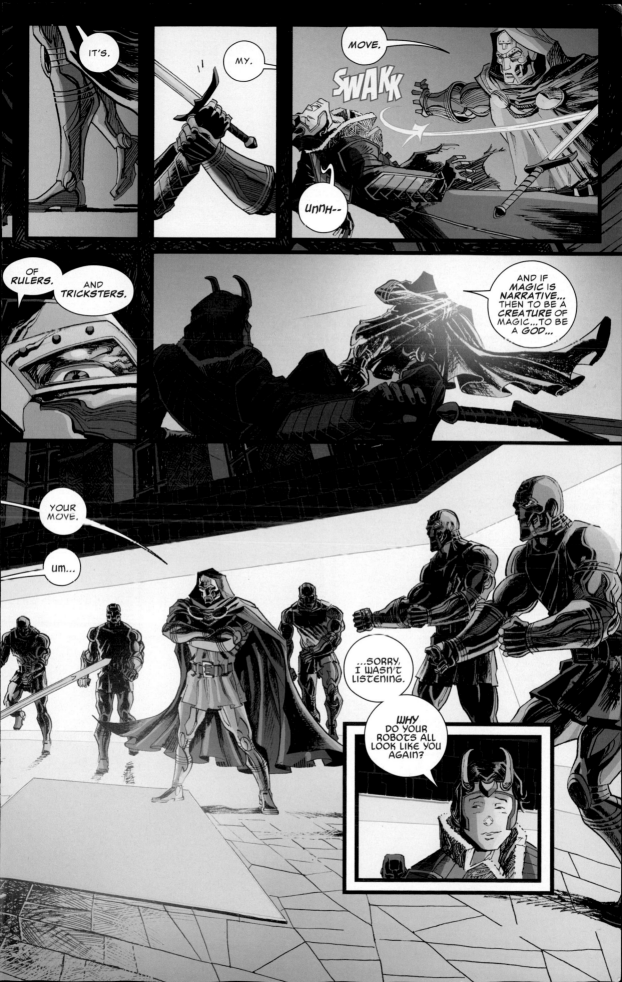

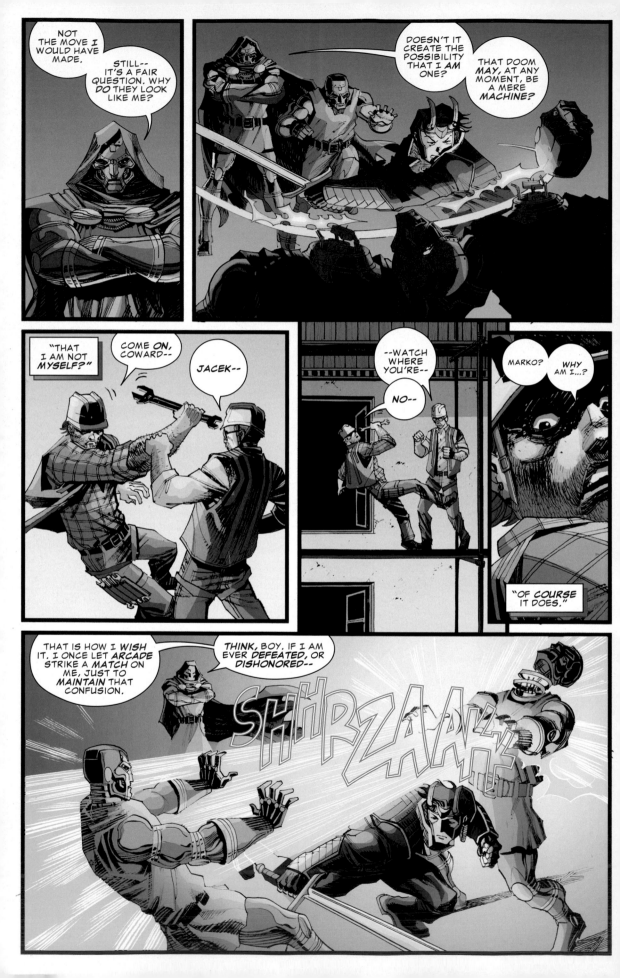

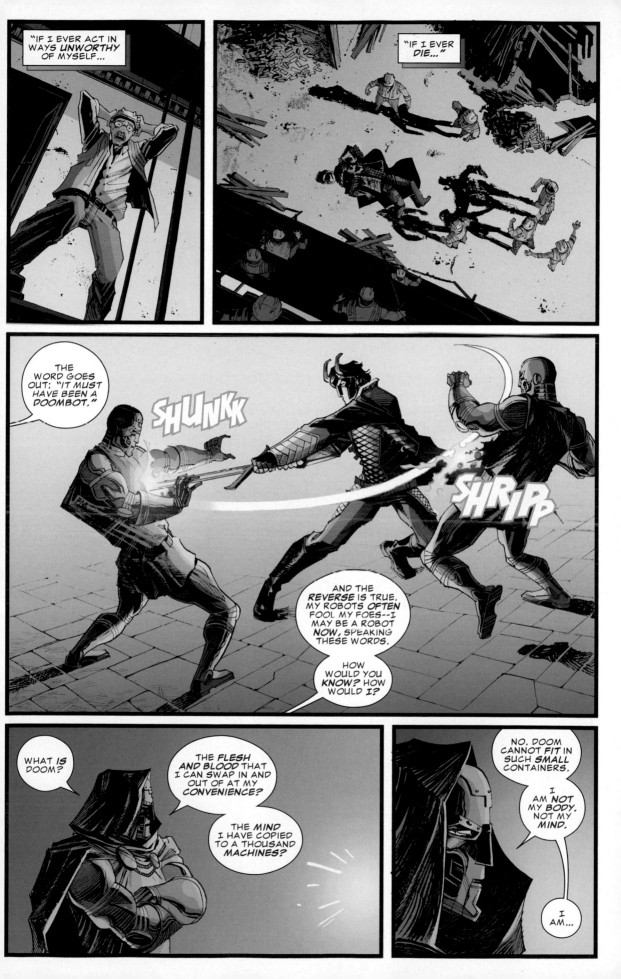

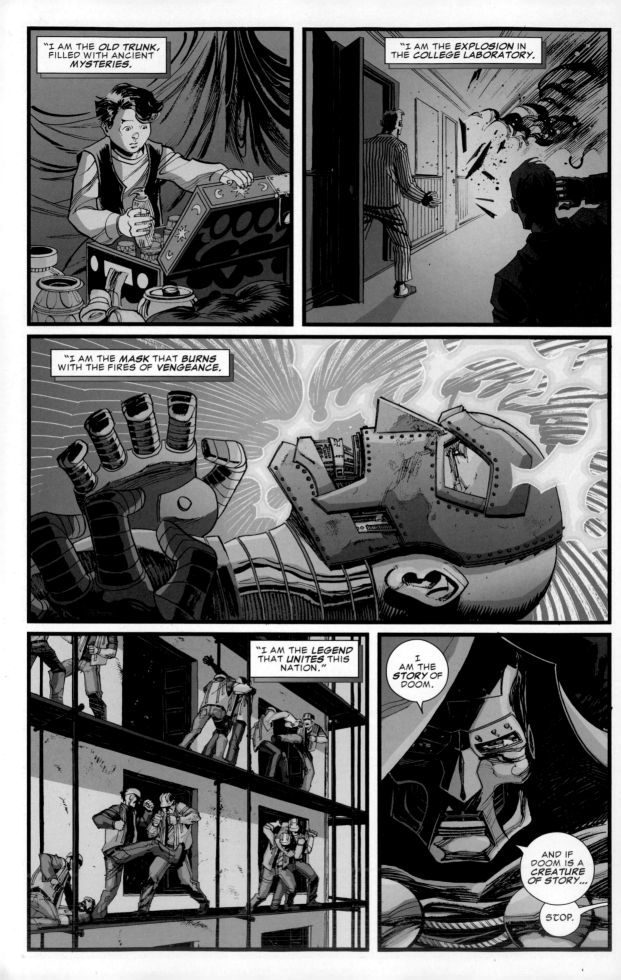

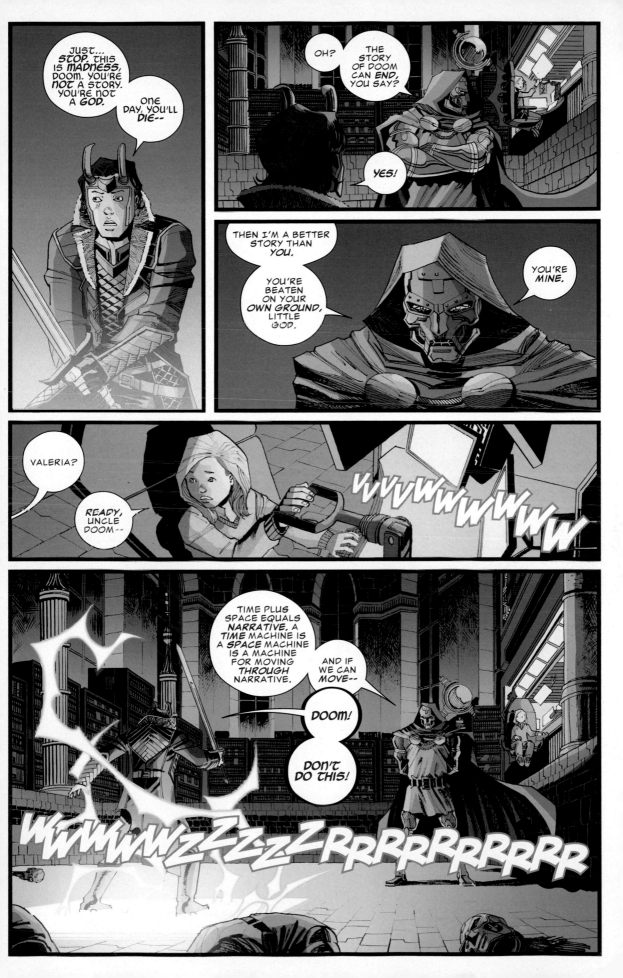

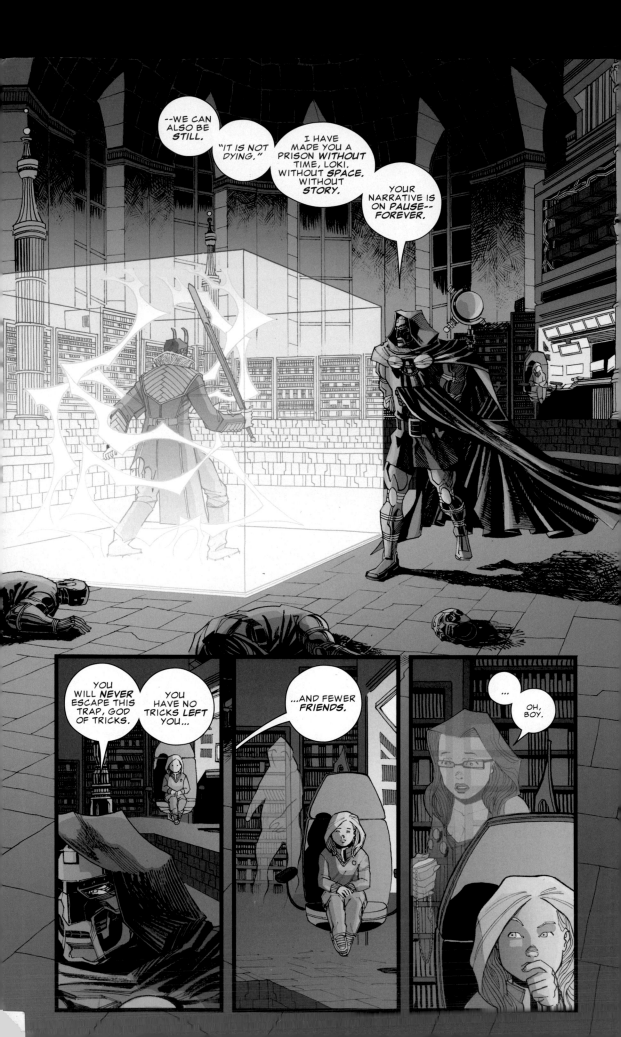

WORLD WAR HATE
HITS LATVERIA!

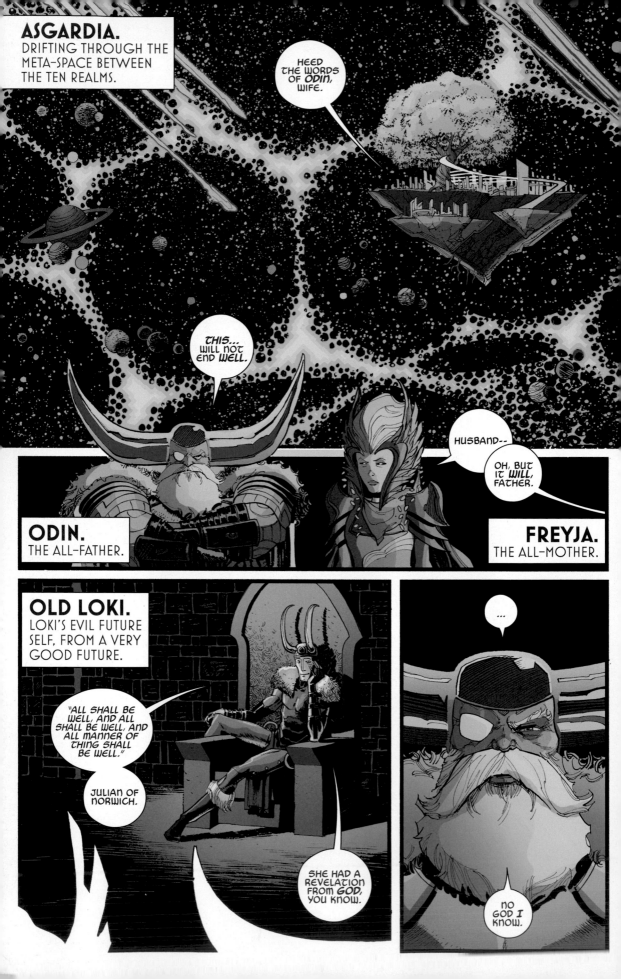

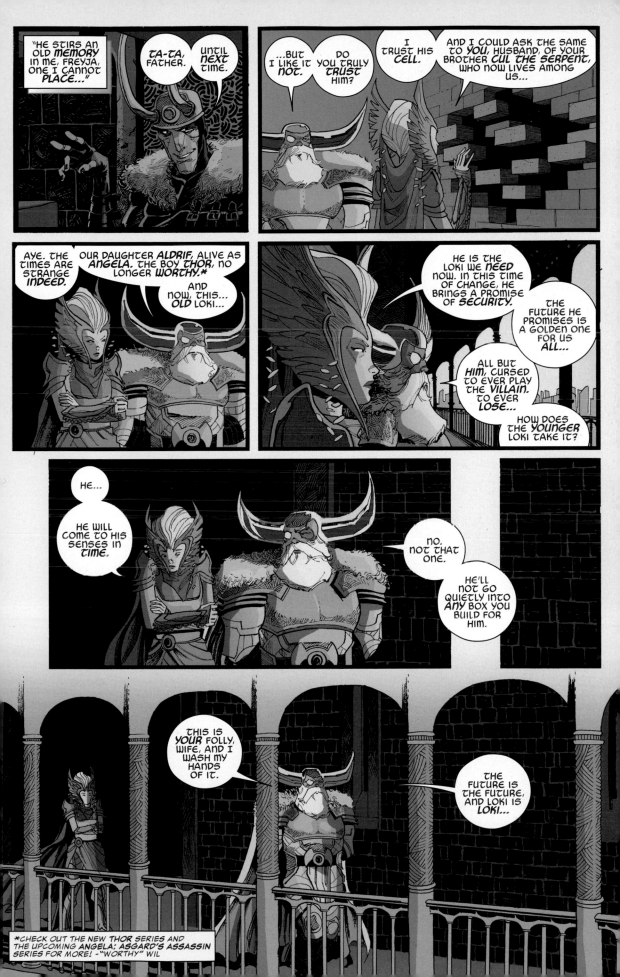

*CHECK OUT THE NEW THOR SERIES AND THE UPCOMING ANGELA: ASGARD'S ASSASSIN SERIES FOR MORE! - "WORTHY" WIL

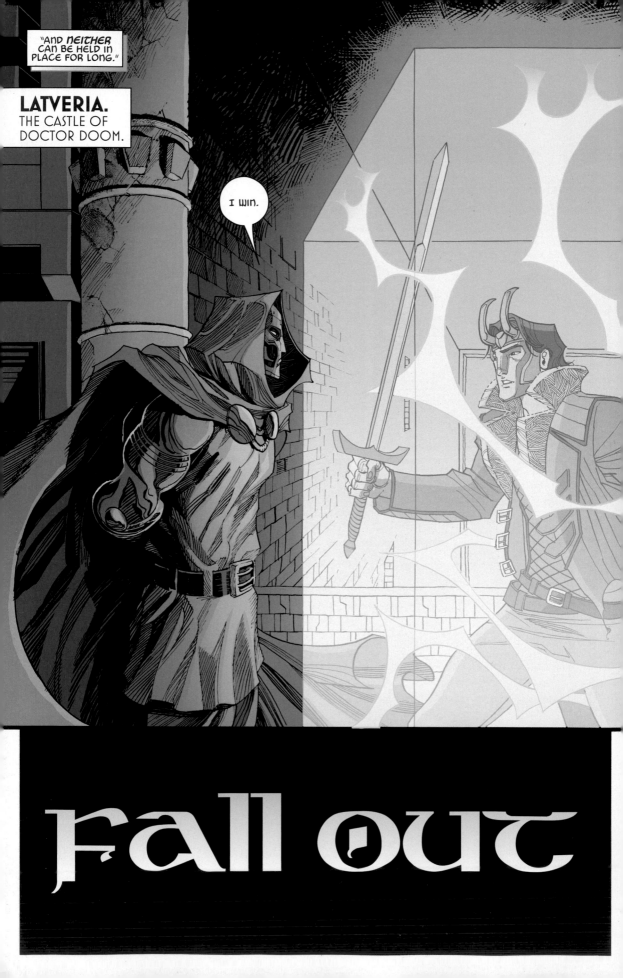

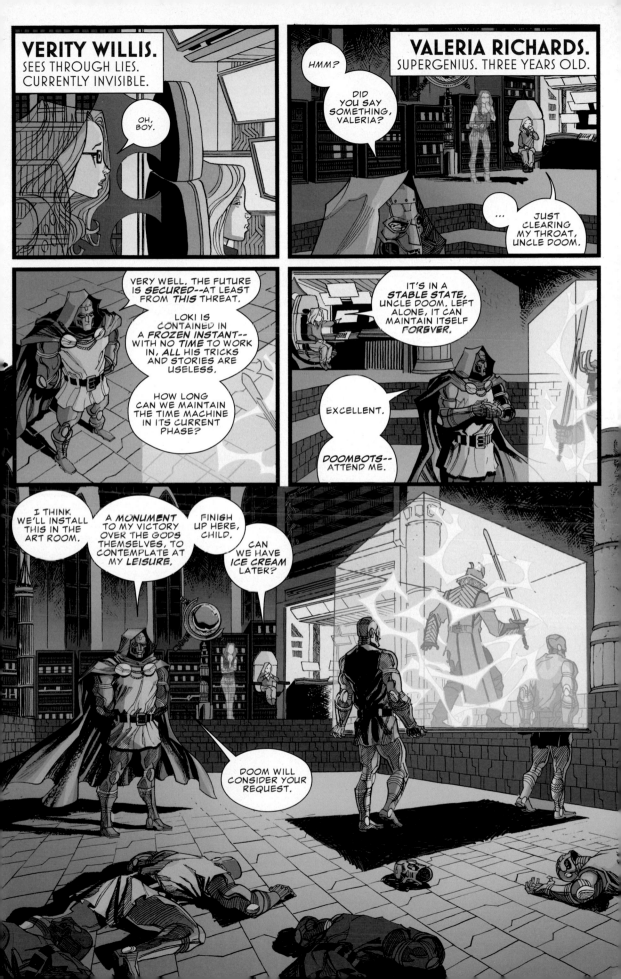

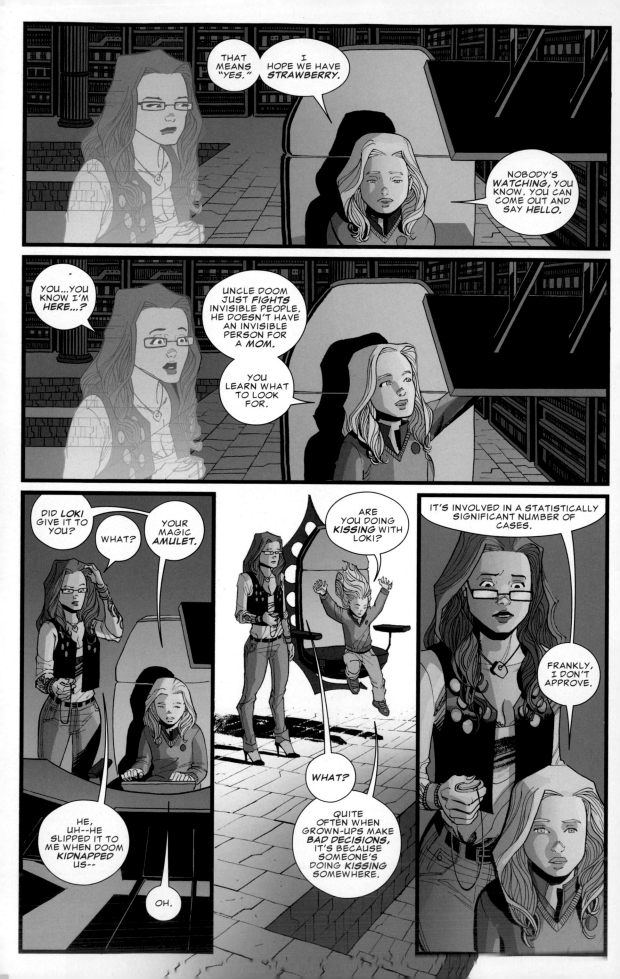

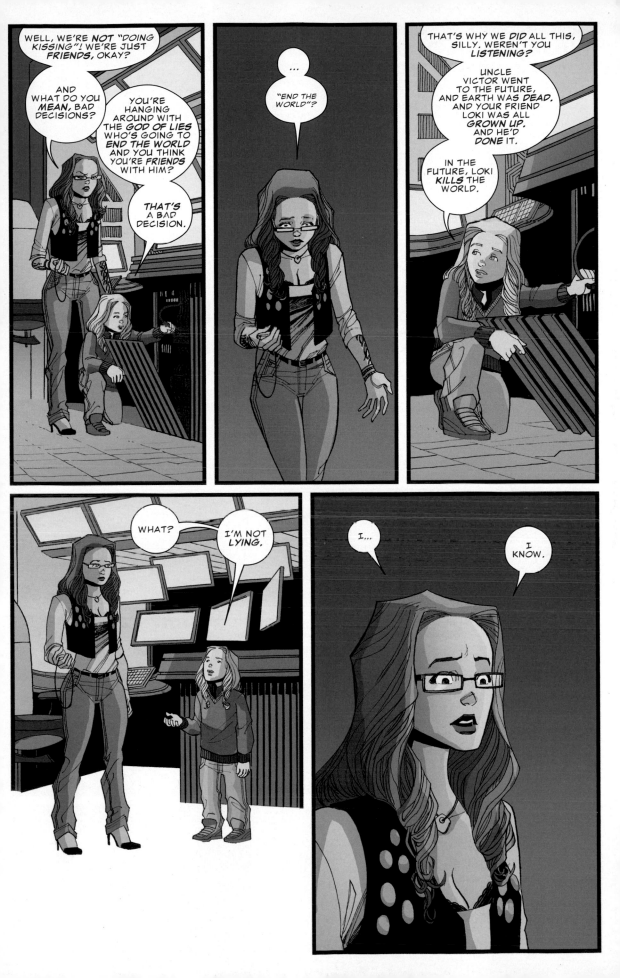

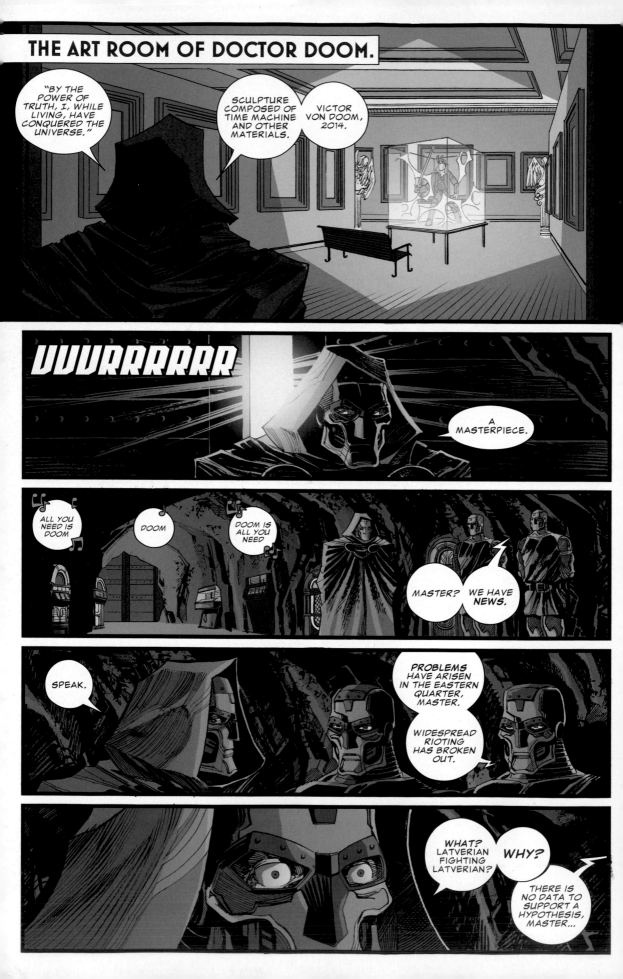

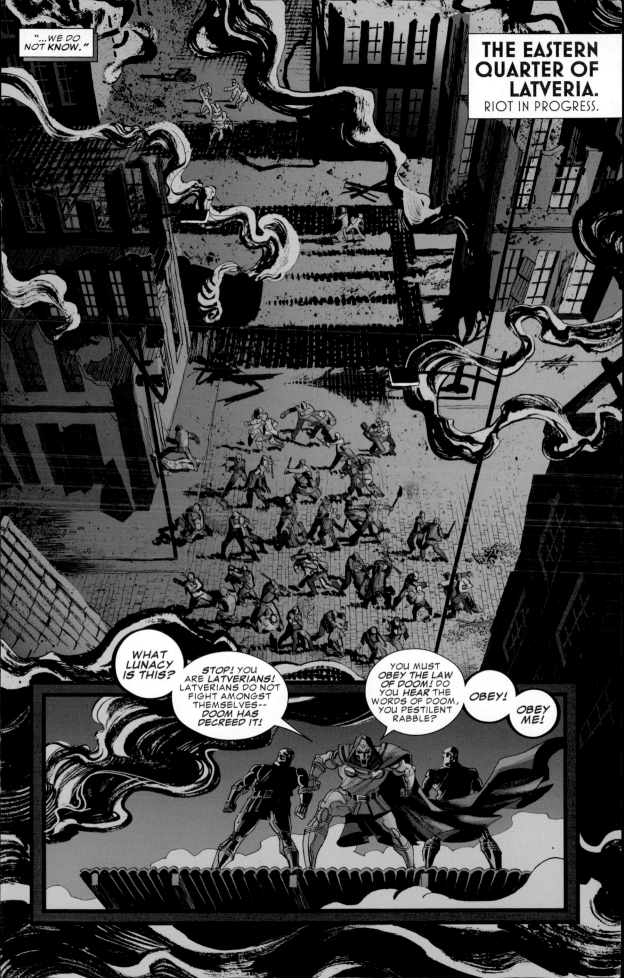

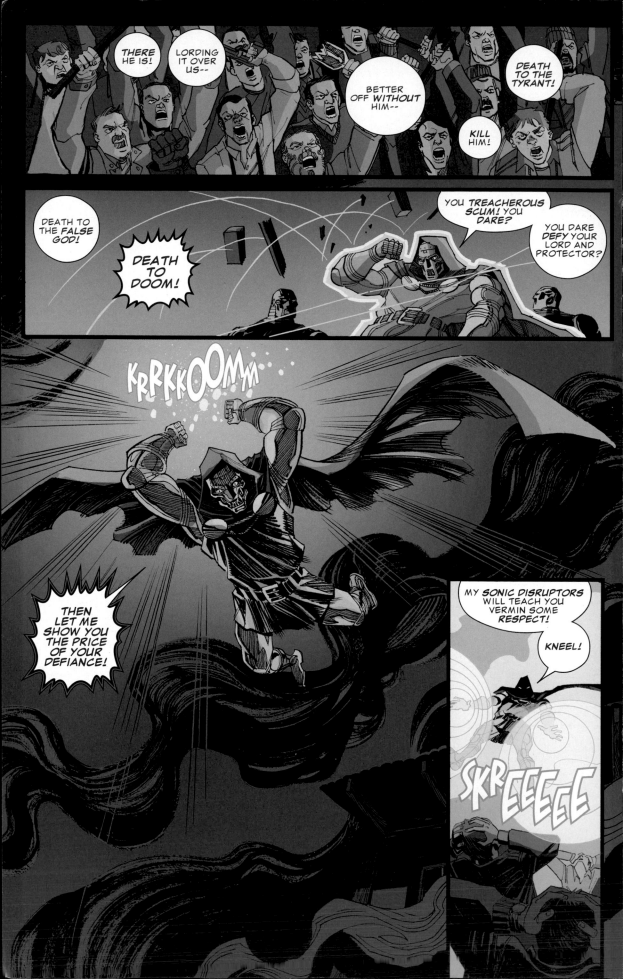

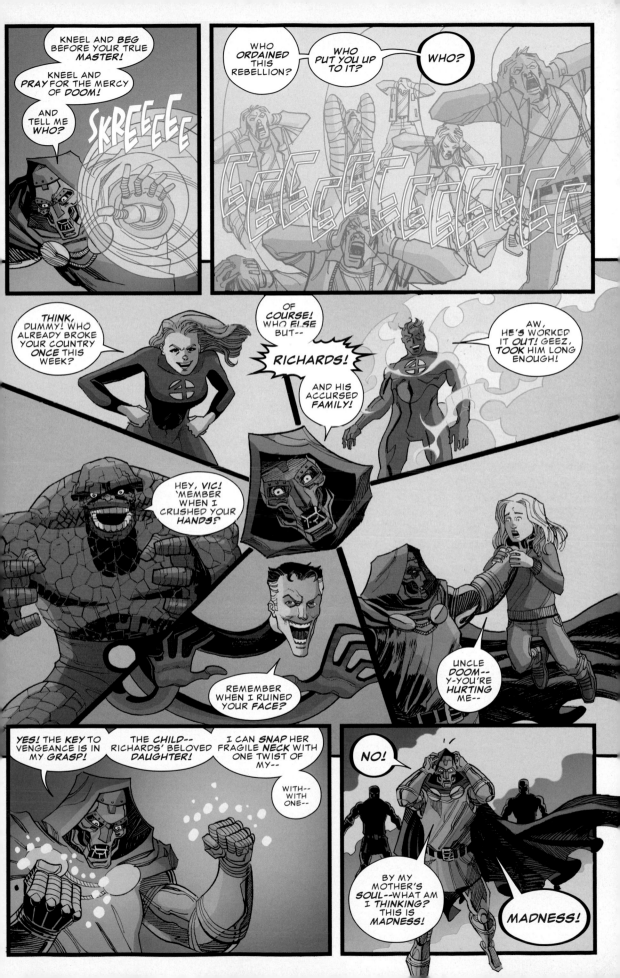

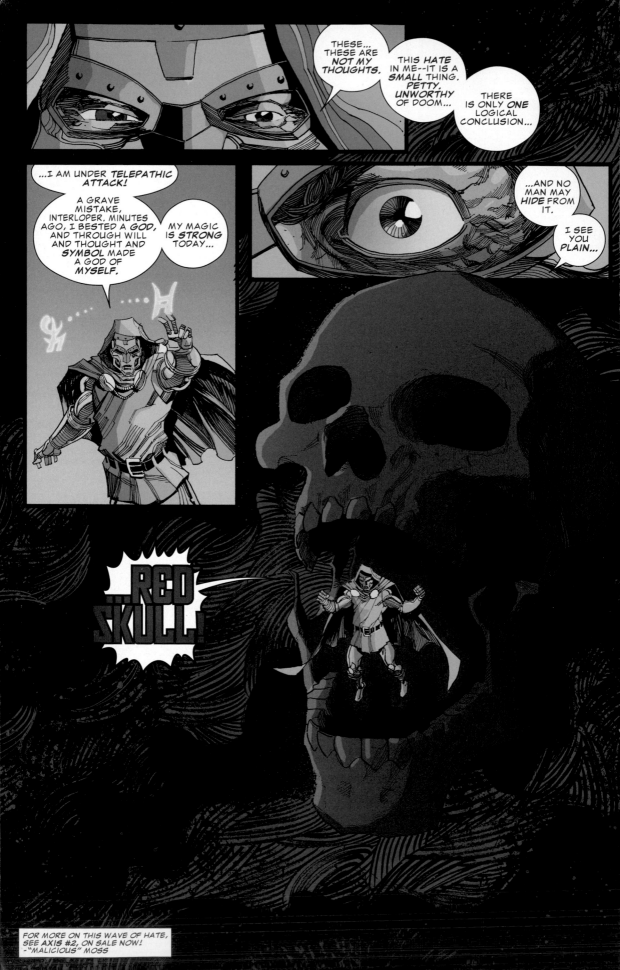

FOR MORE ON THIS WAVE OF HATE, SEE AXIS #2, ON SALE NOW! -"MALICIOUS" MOSS

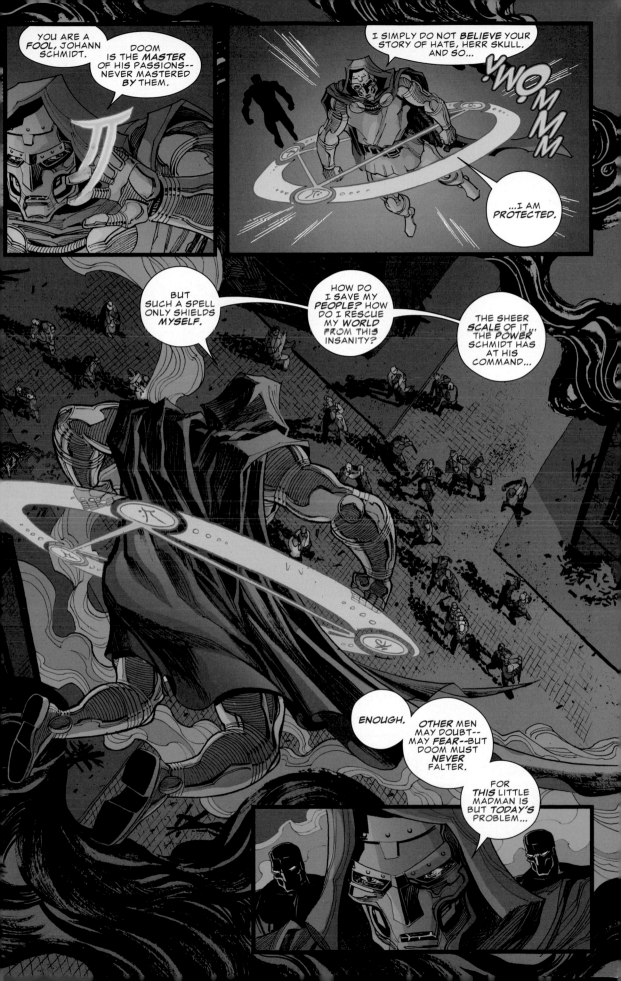

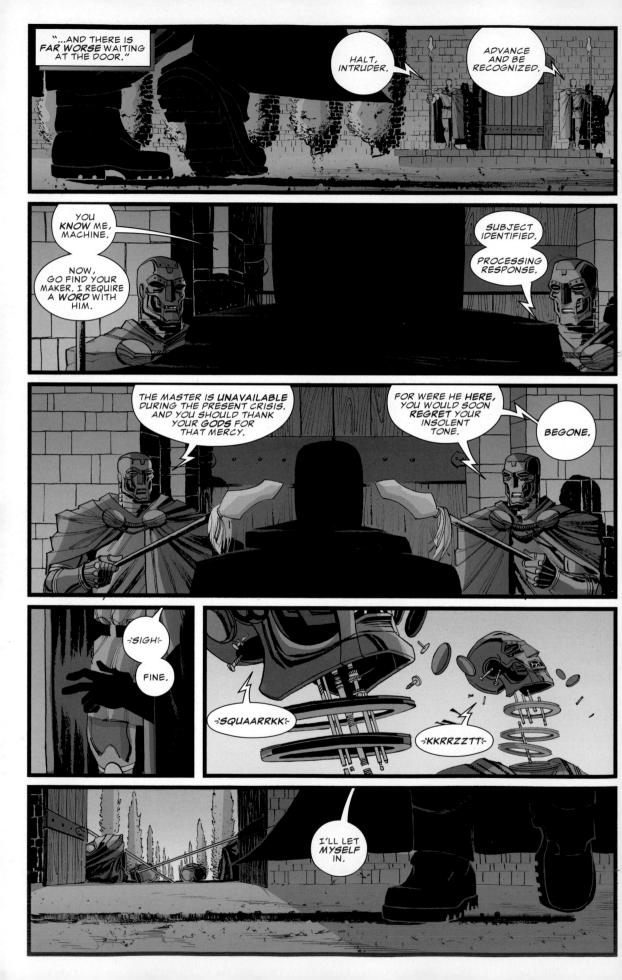

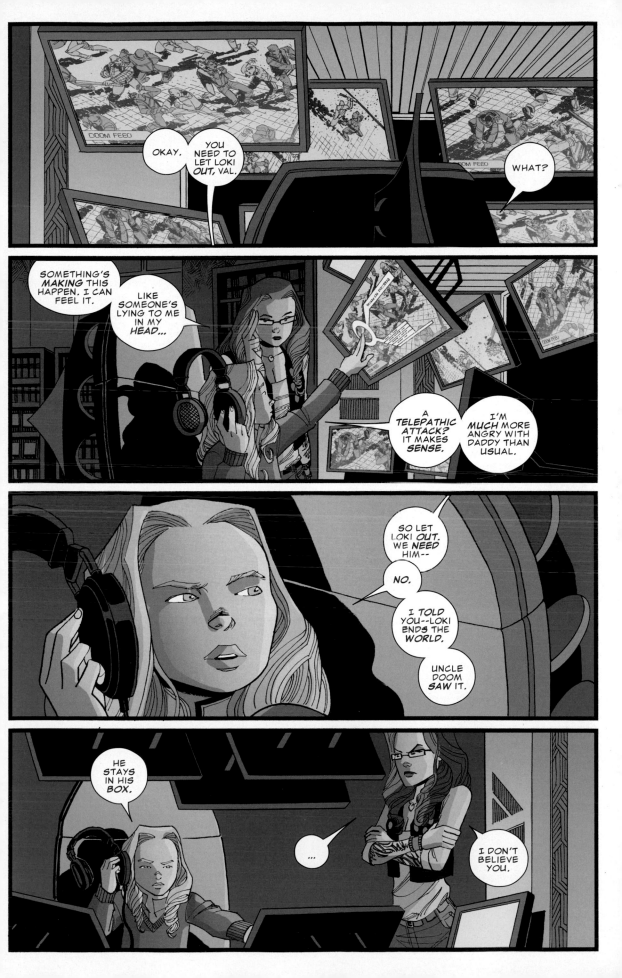

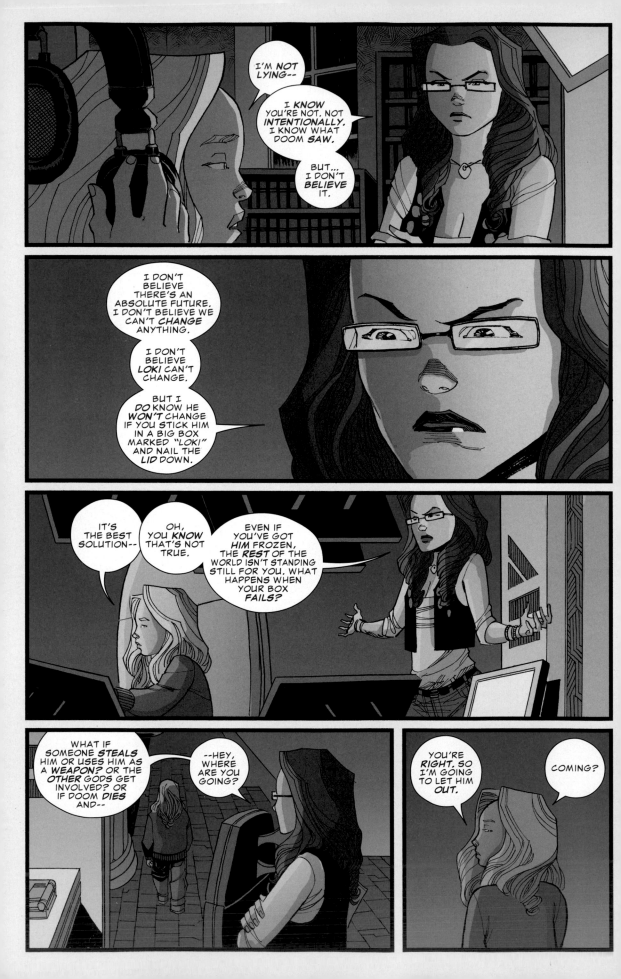

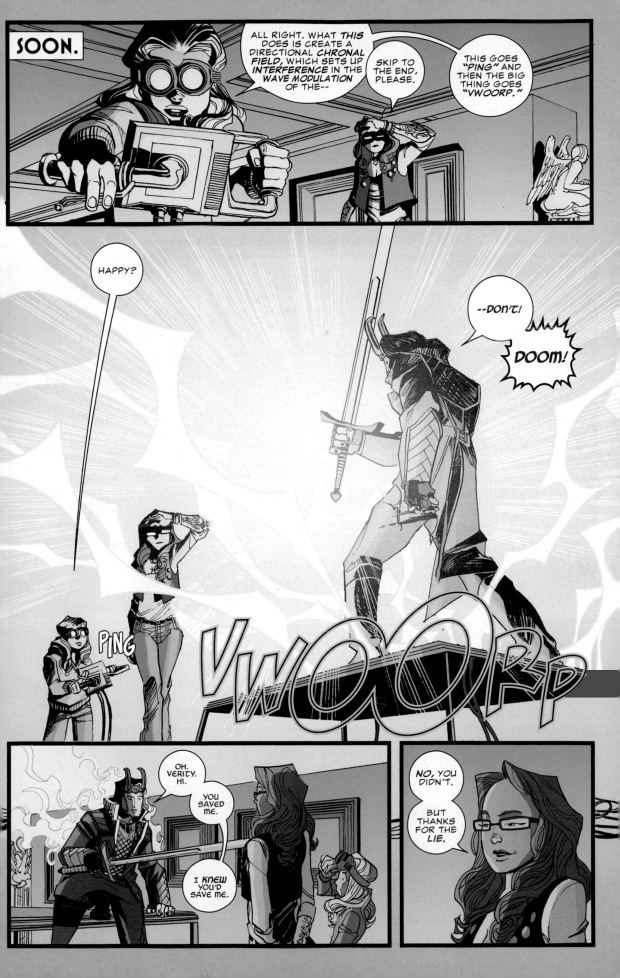

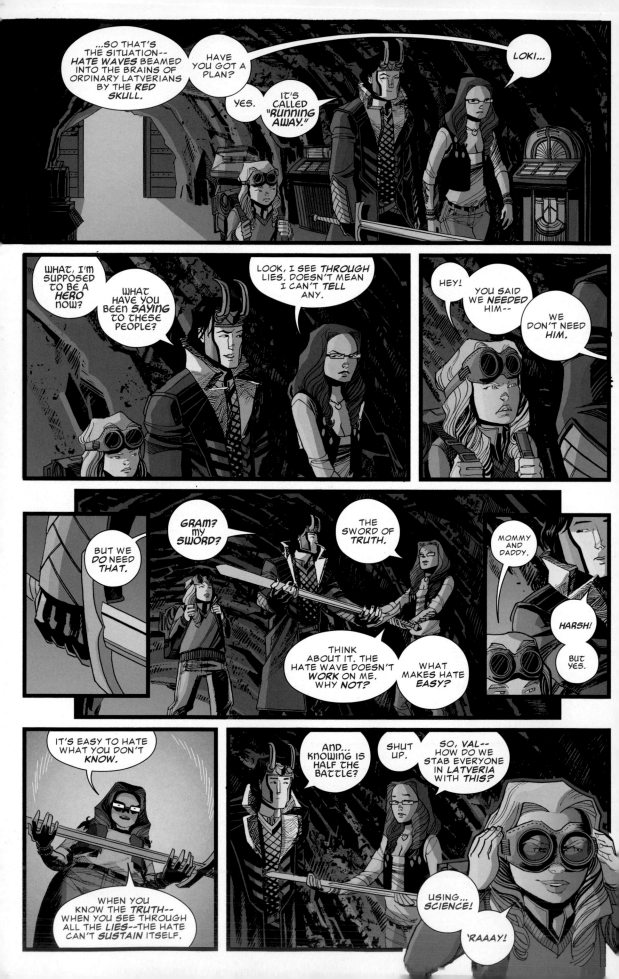

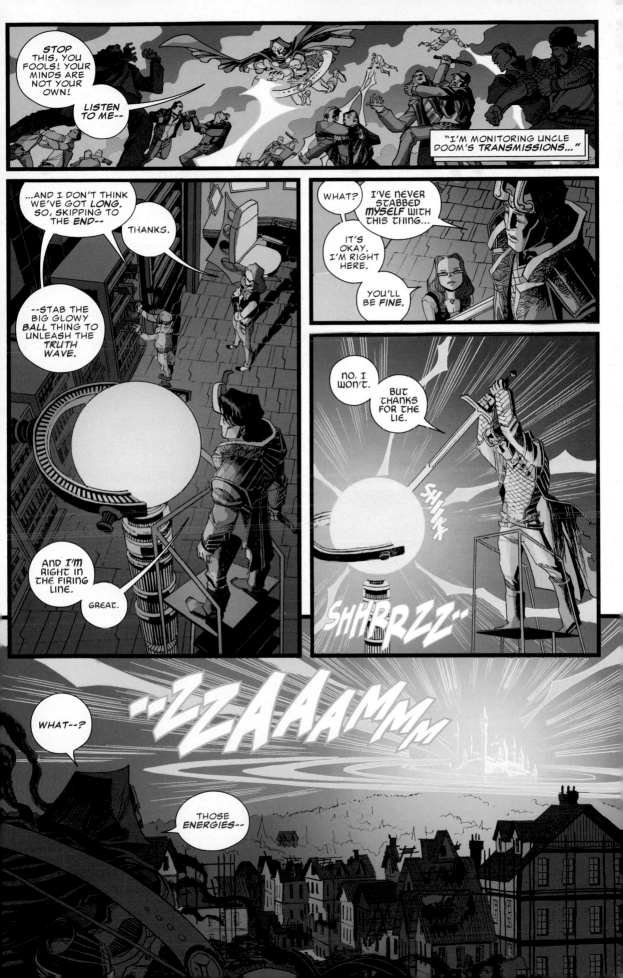

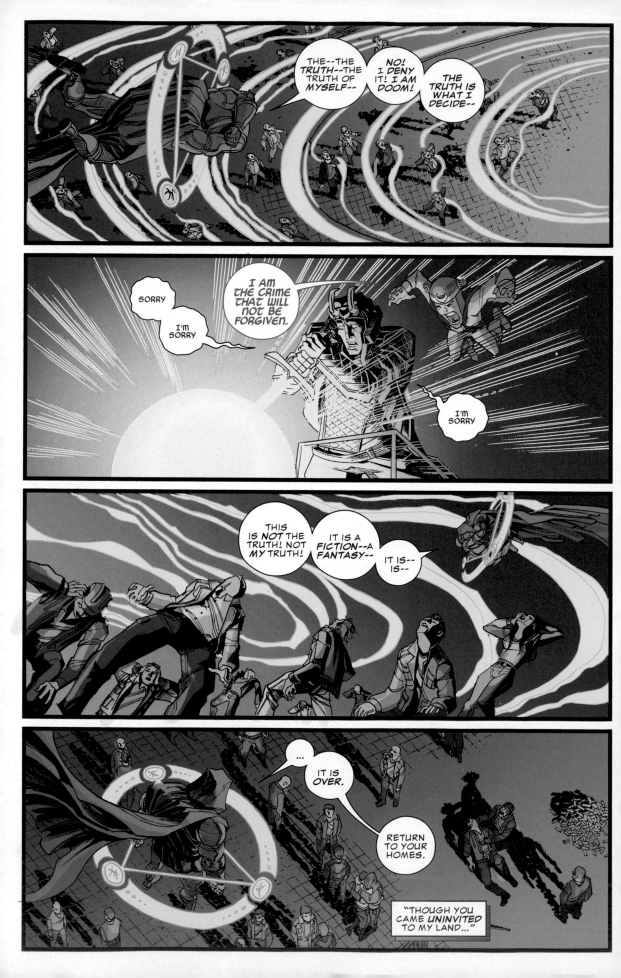

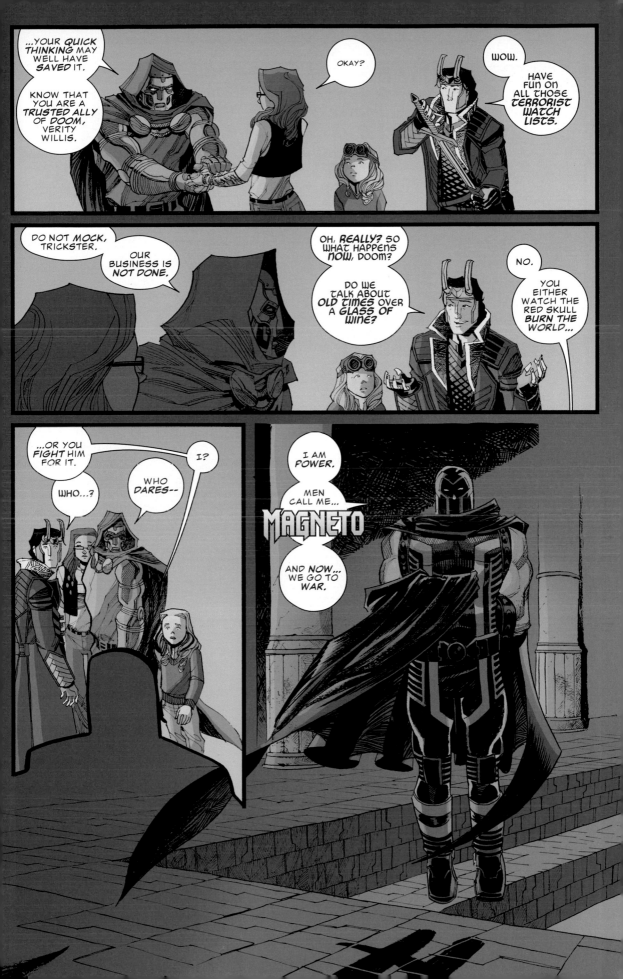

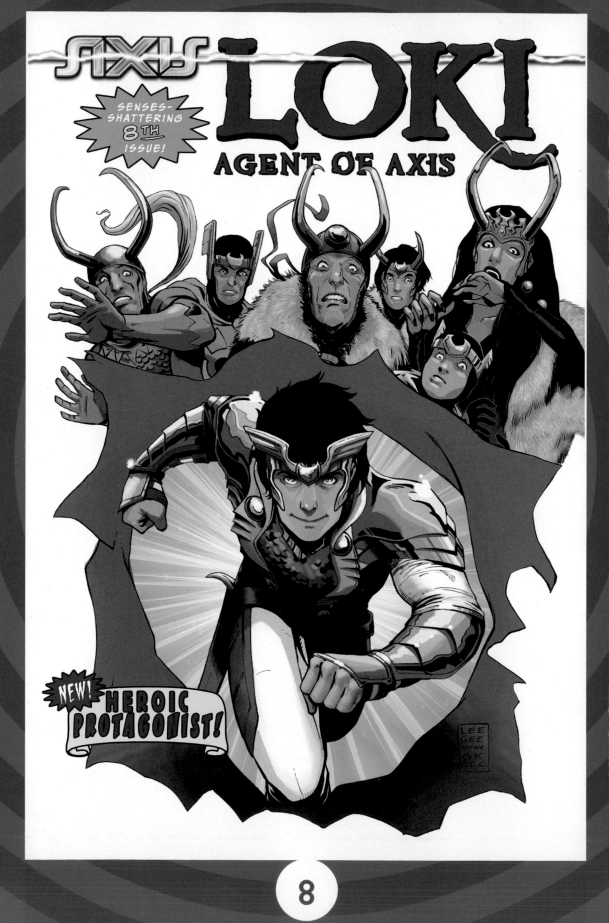

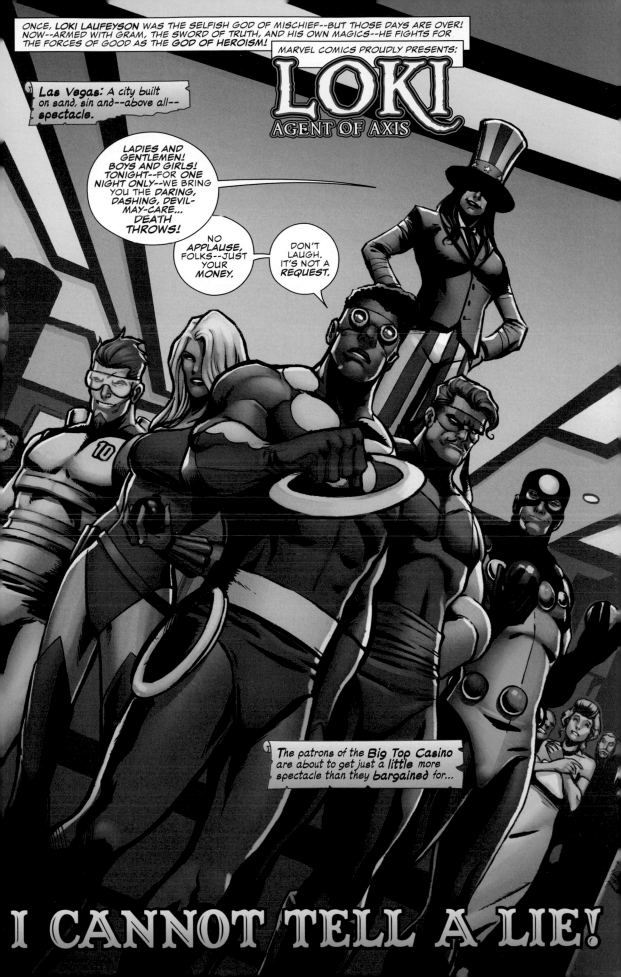

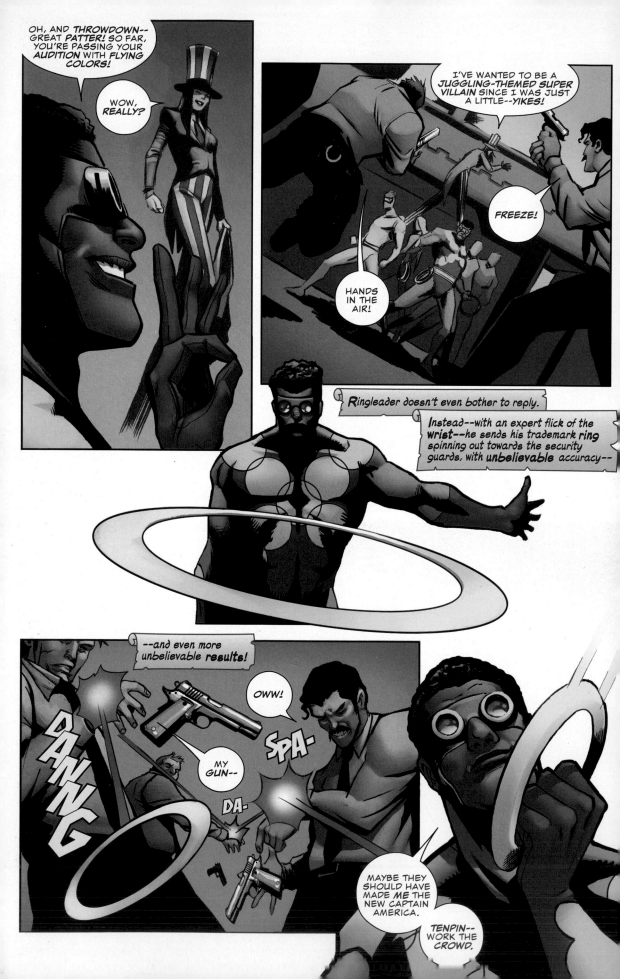

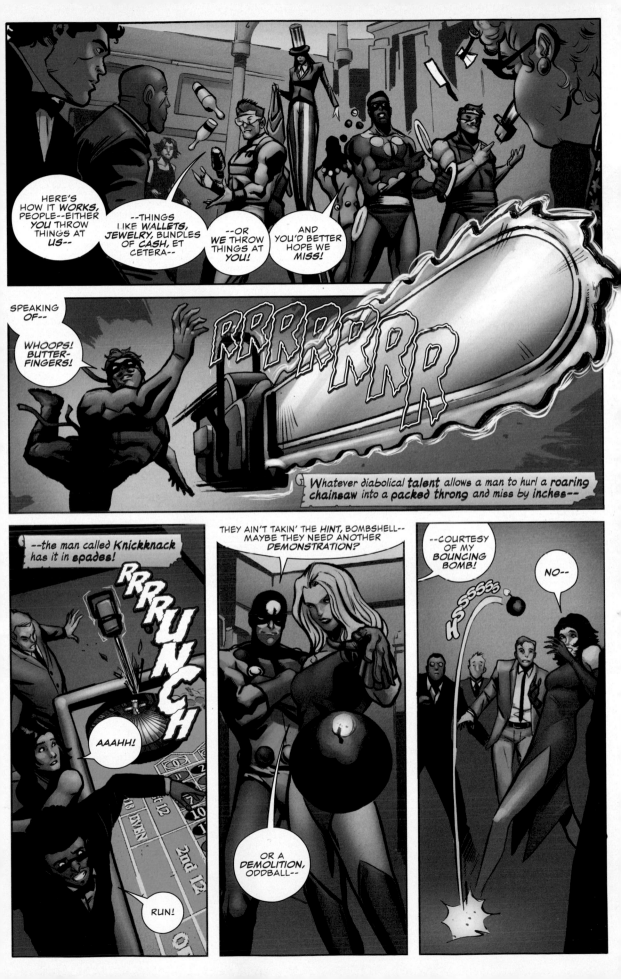

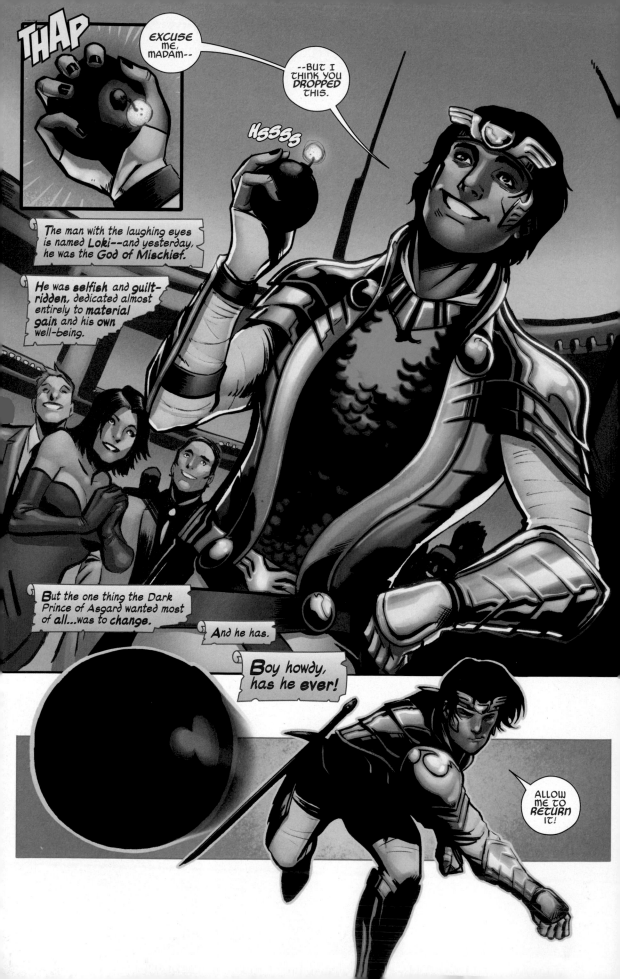

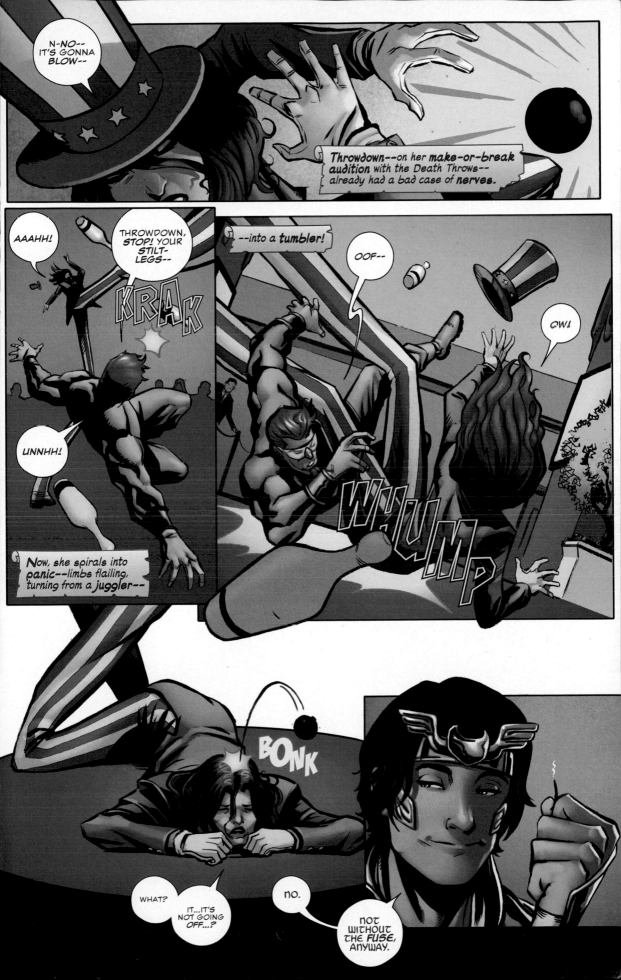

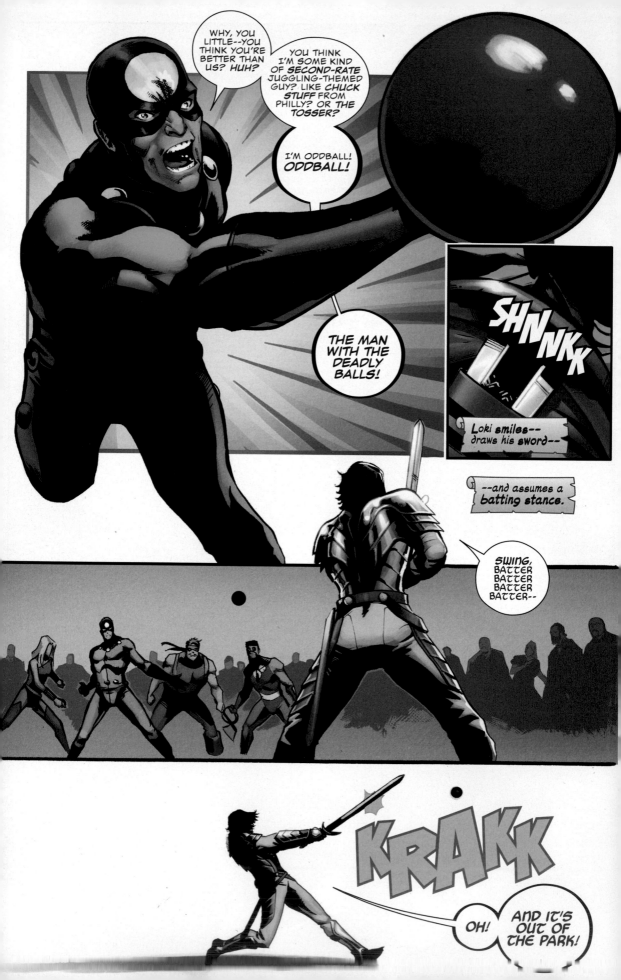

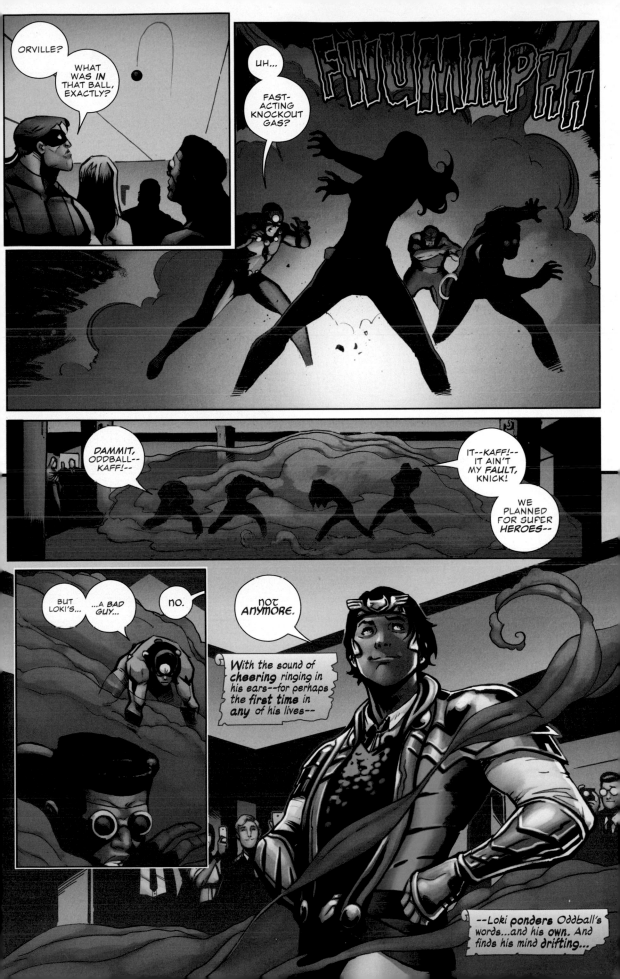

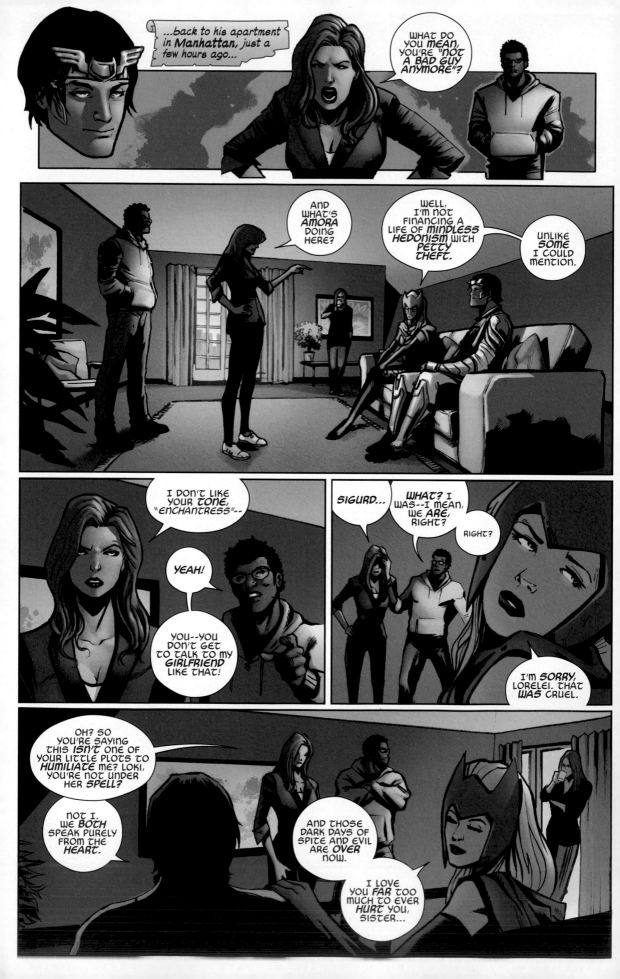

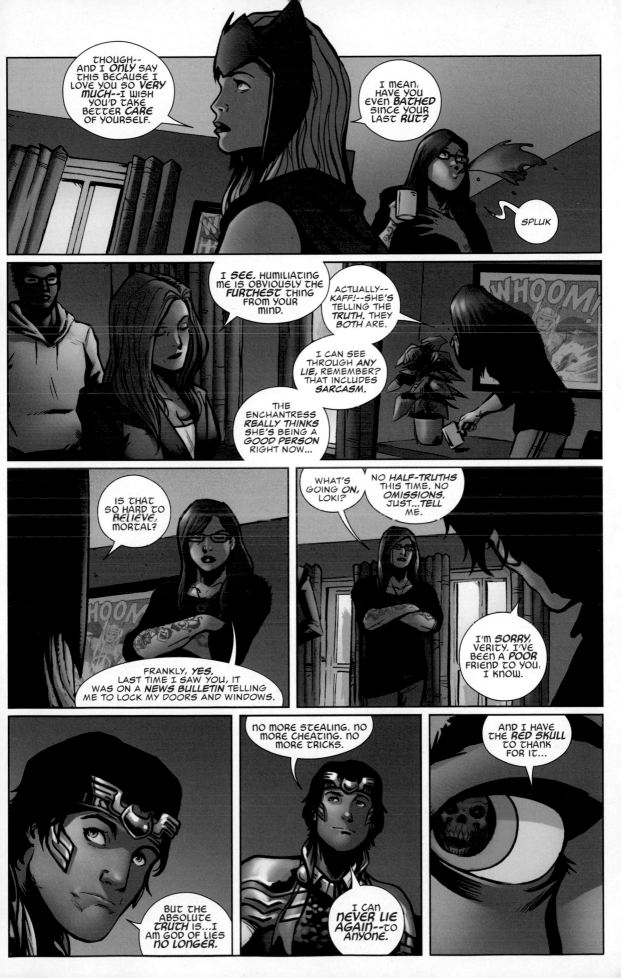

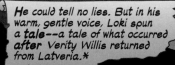

He could tell no lies. But in his warm, gentle voice, Loki spun a *tale*—a tale of what occurred *after* Verity Willis returned from Latveria.*

A tale of the *final battle* between the *Red Skull* and a *loose coalition* of *super villains*, fighting alongside the heroes for their *own* lives and freedoms...

A tale of a fateful *spell*, cast by the Scarlet Witch and Doctor Doom, mixing *order* and *chaos* to defeat the Skull once and for all...

*AFTER THE EVENTS OF LAST ISSUE! -WIL

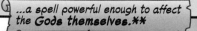

...a spell powerful enough to affect the Gods themselves.**

**READ THE FULL STORY IN THE NOW-CLASSIC *AXIS* #3, TRUE BELIEVER! -WIL

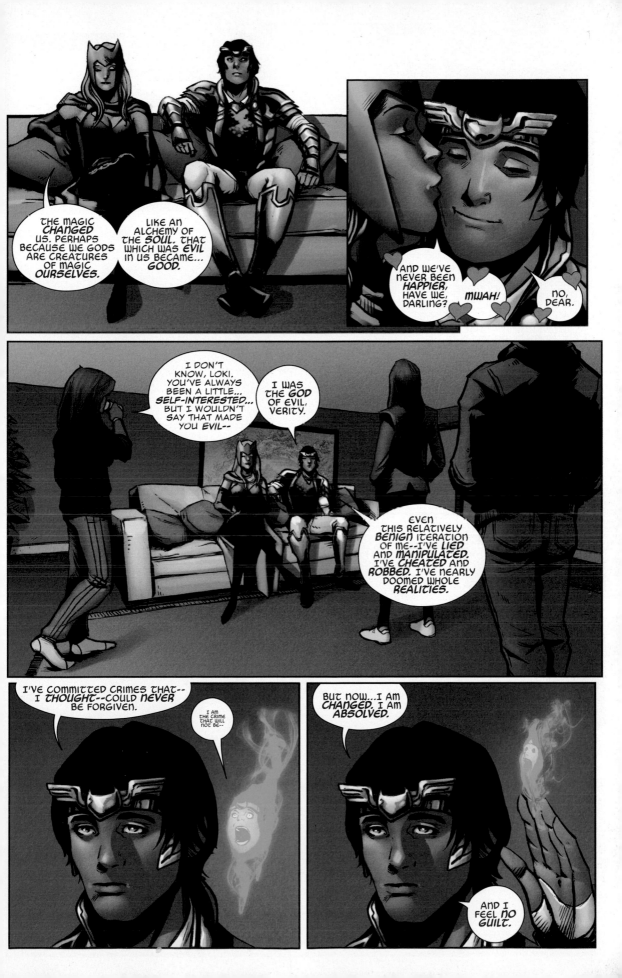

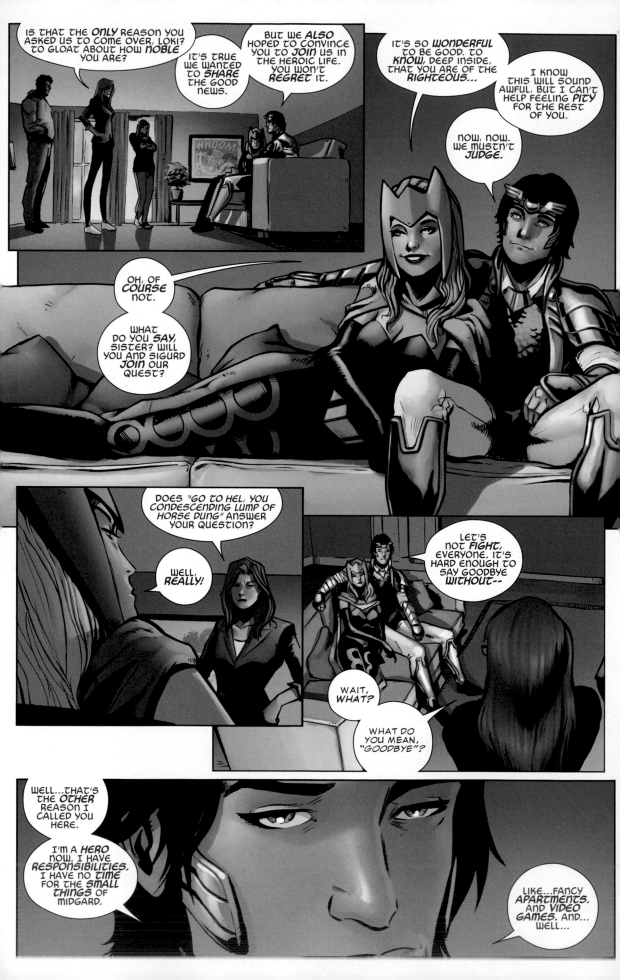

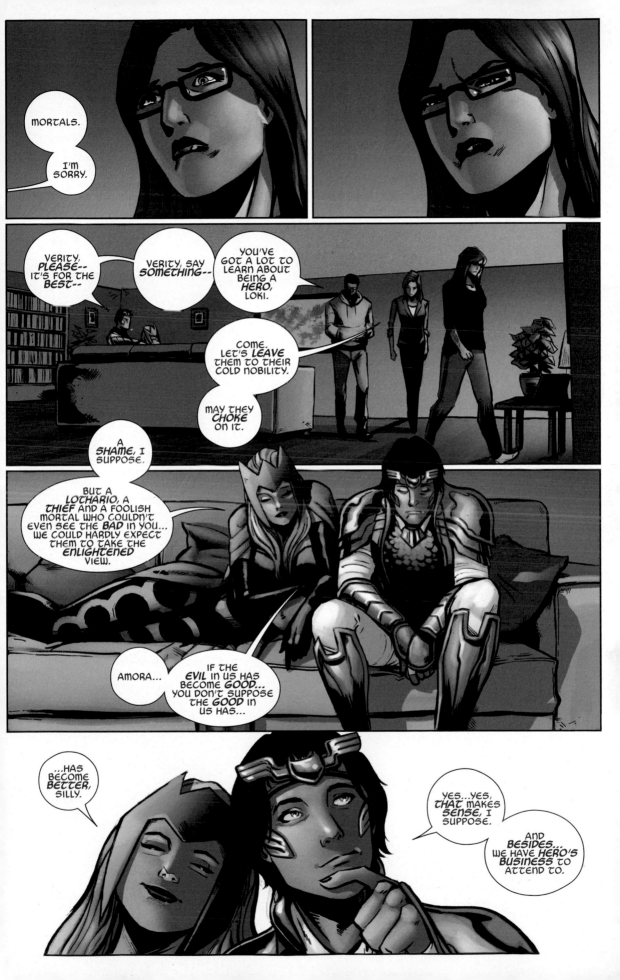

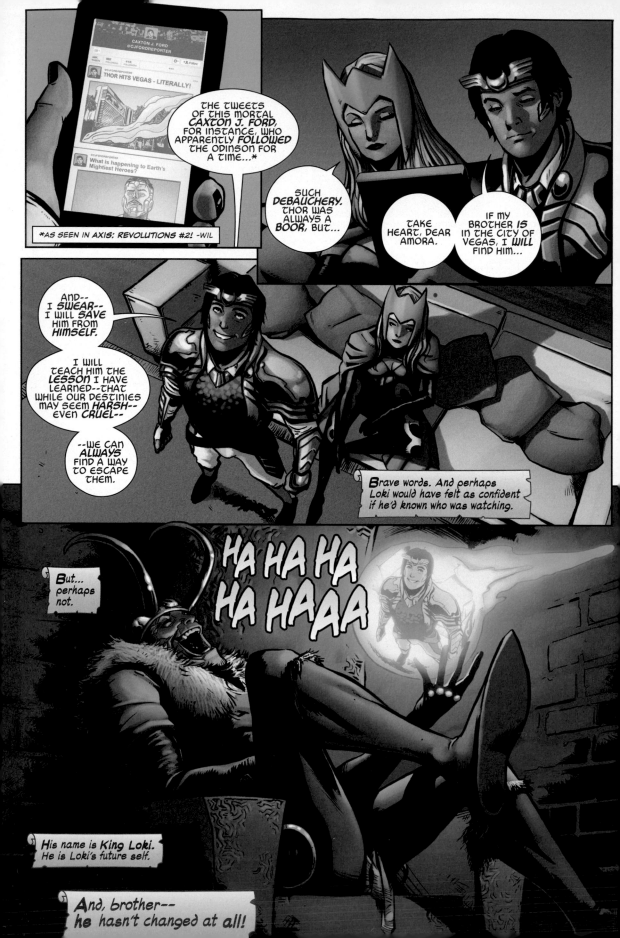

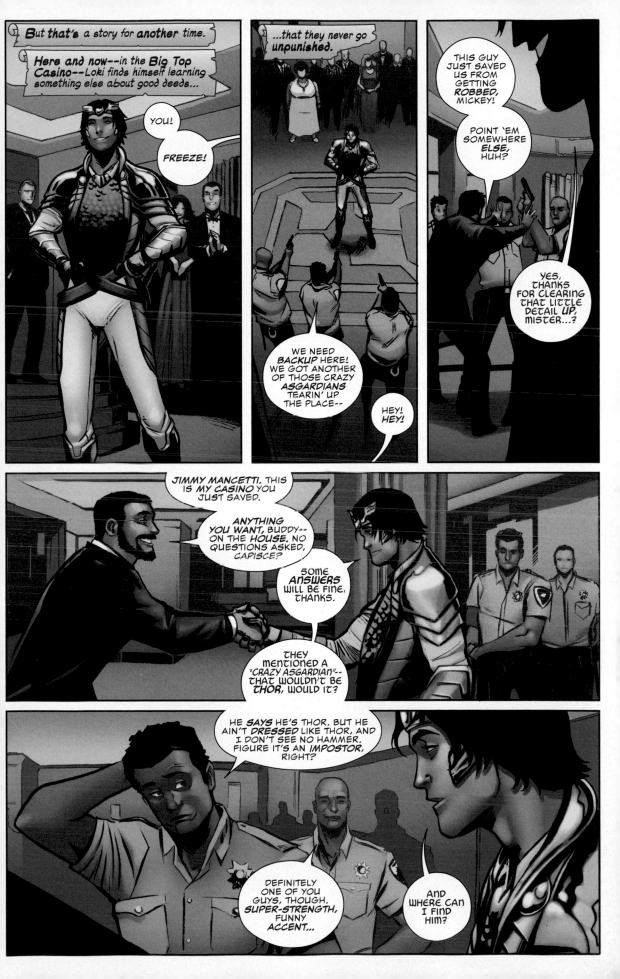

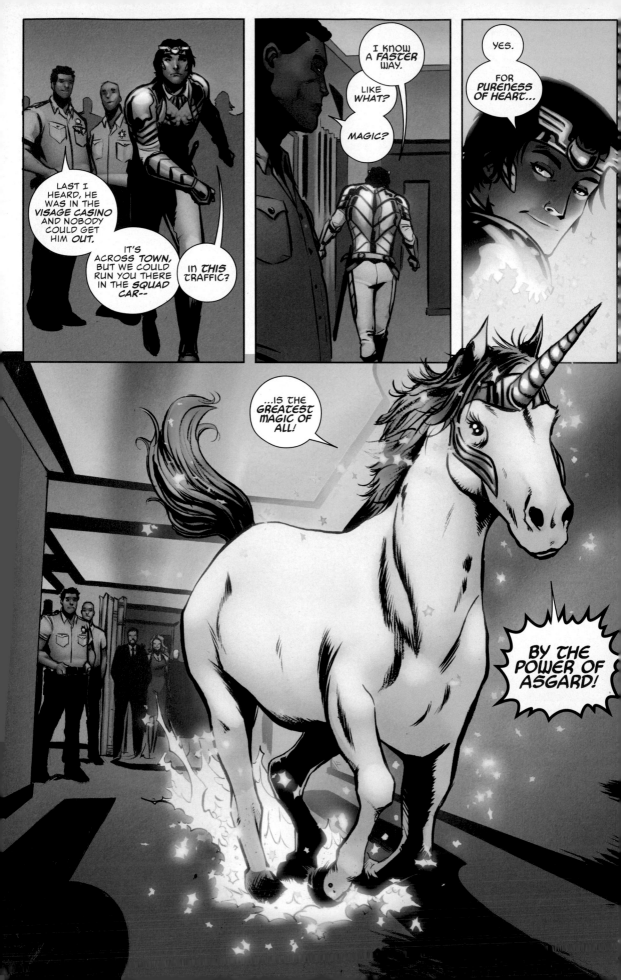

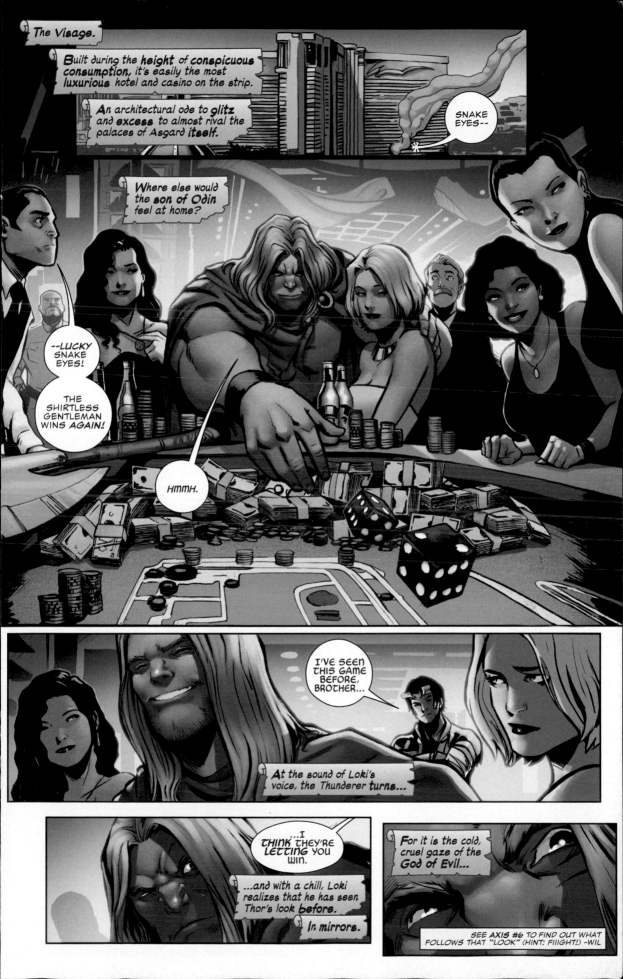

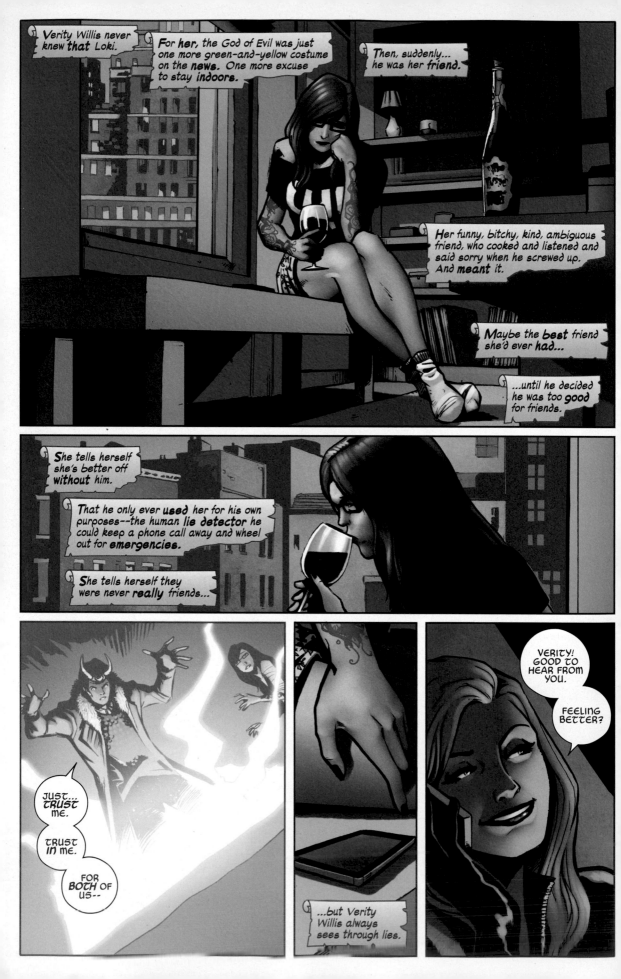

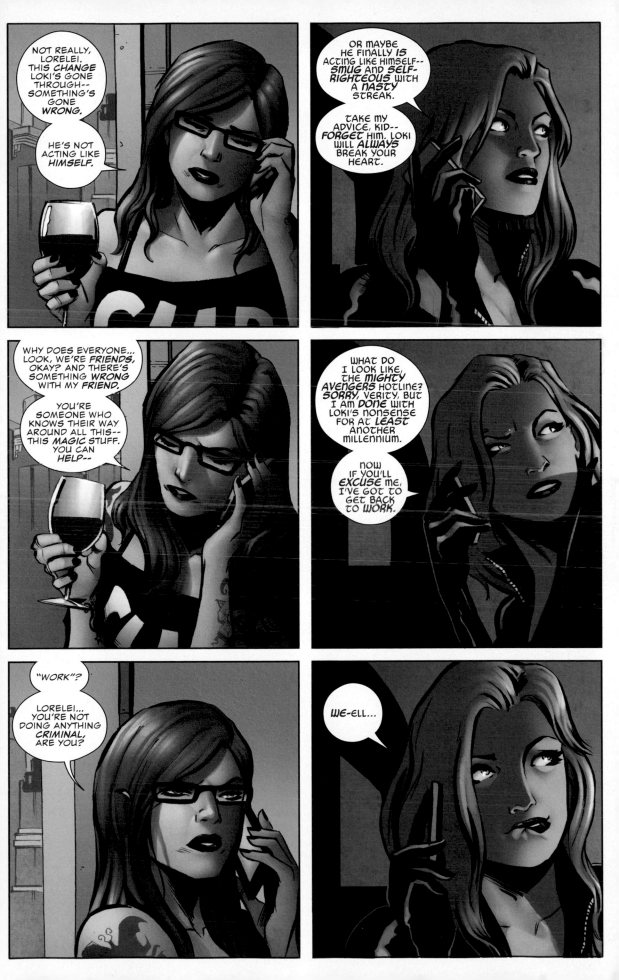

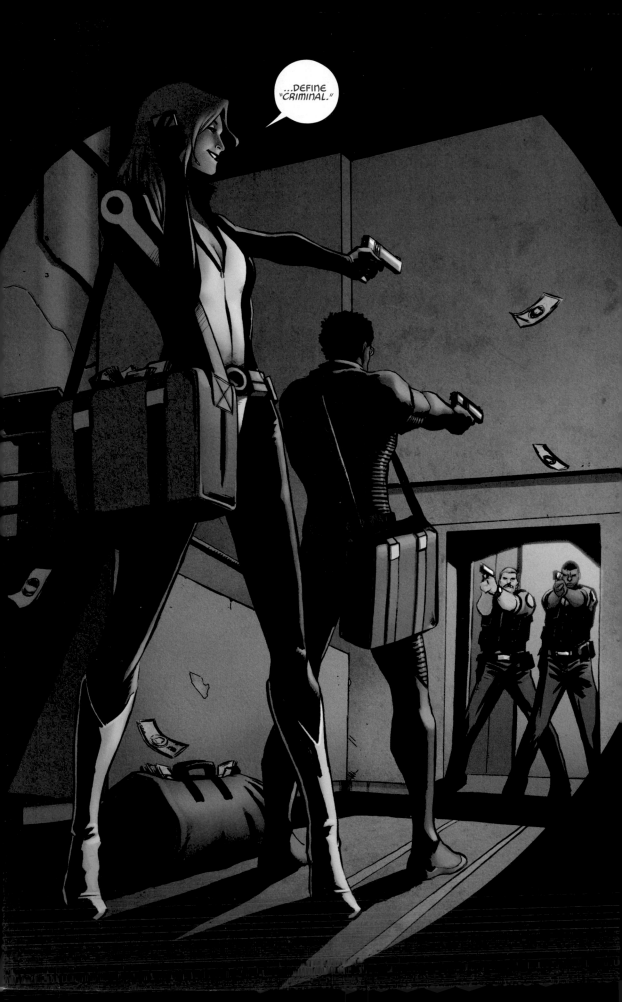

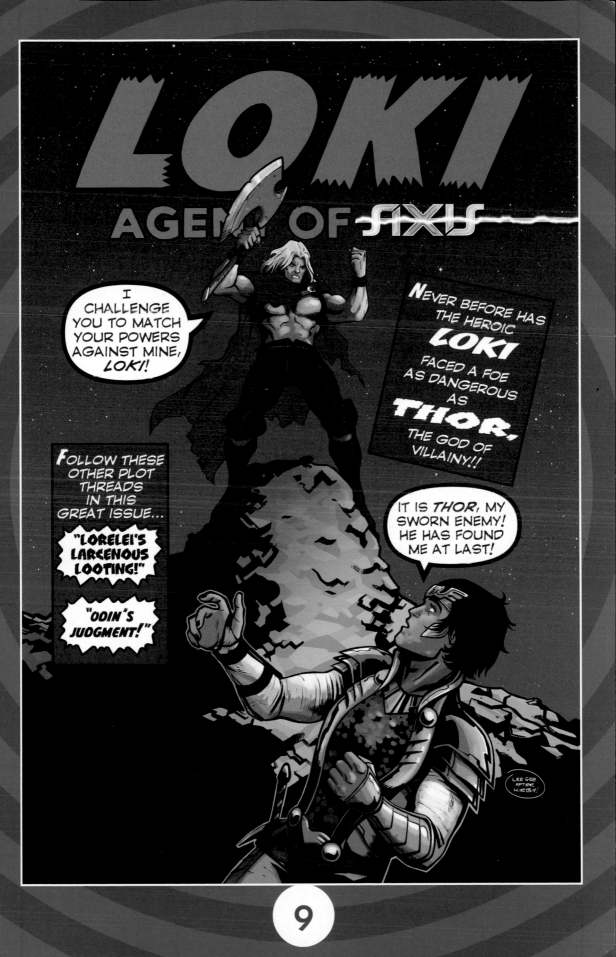

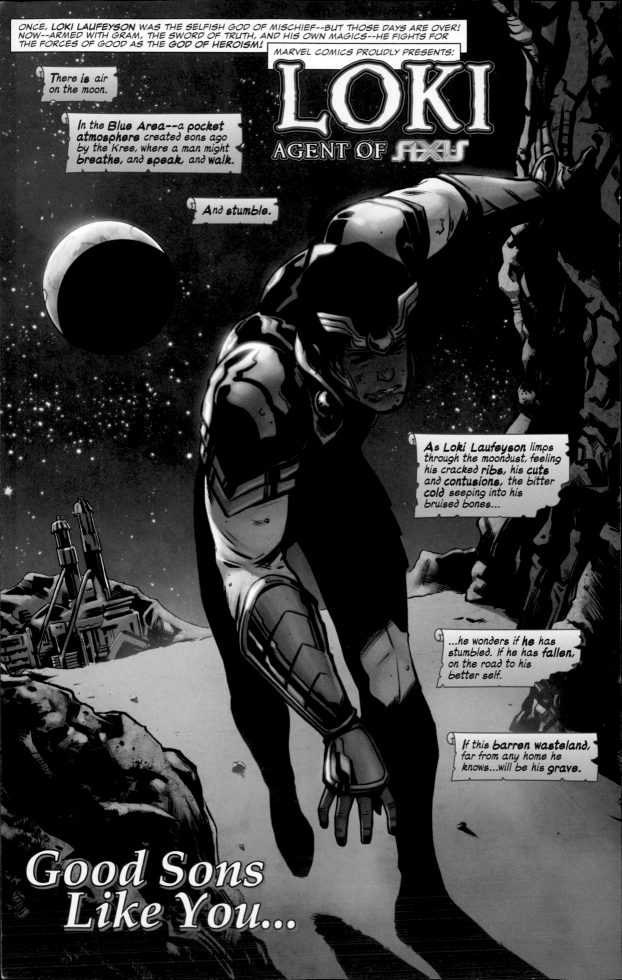

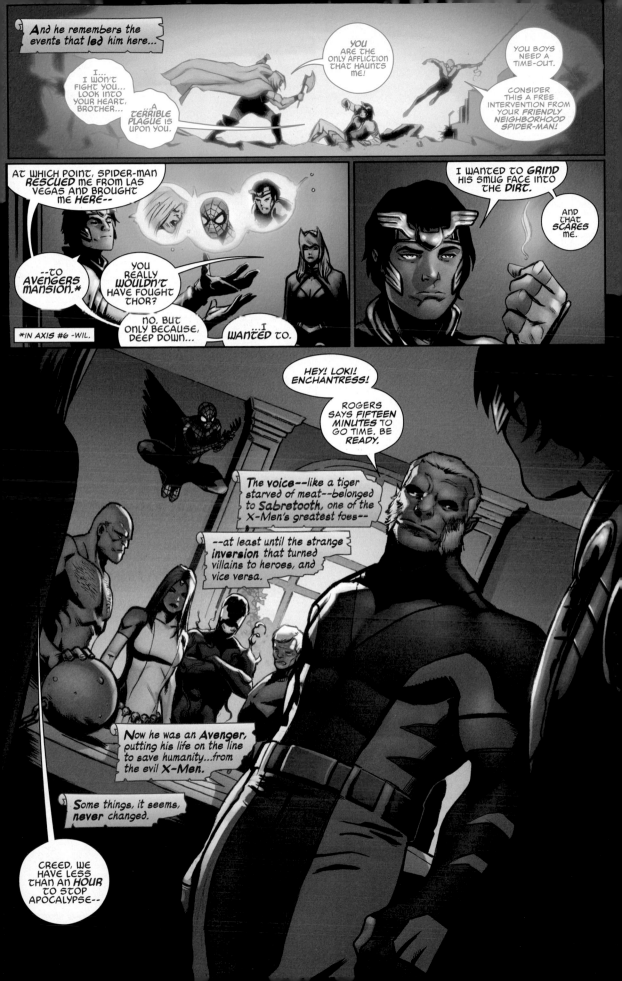

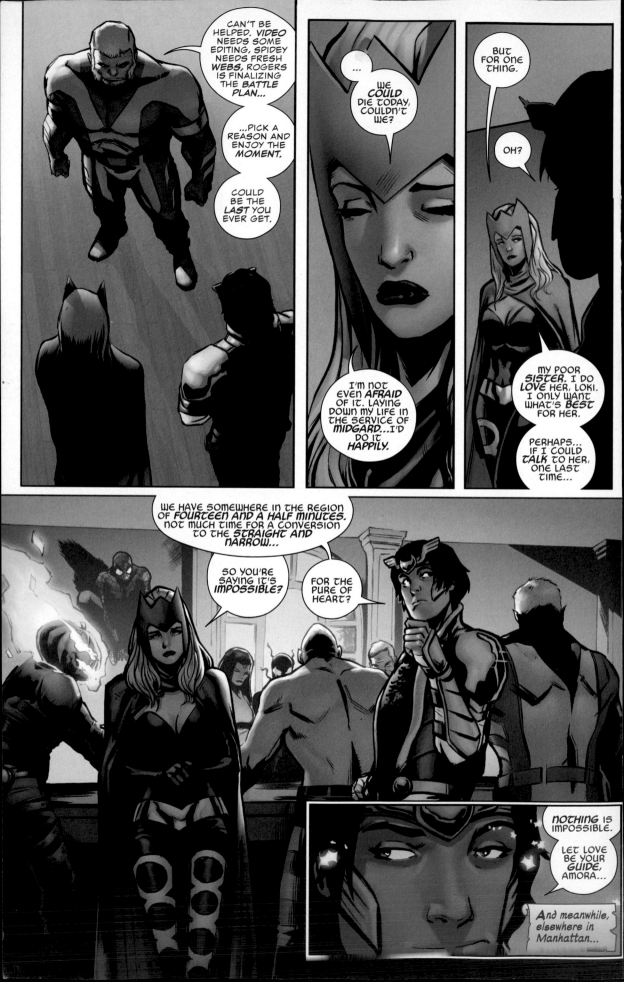

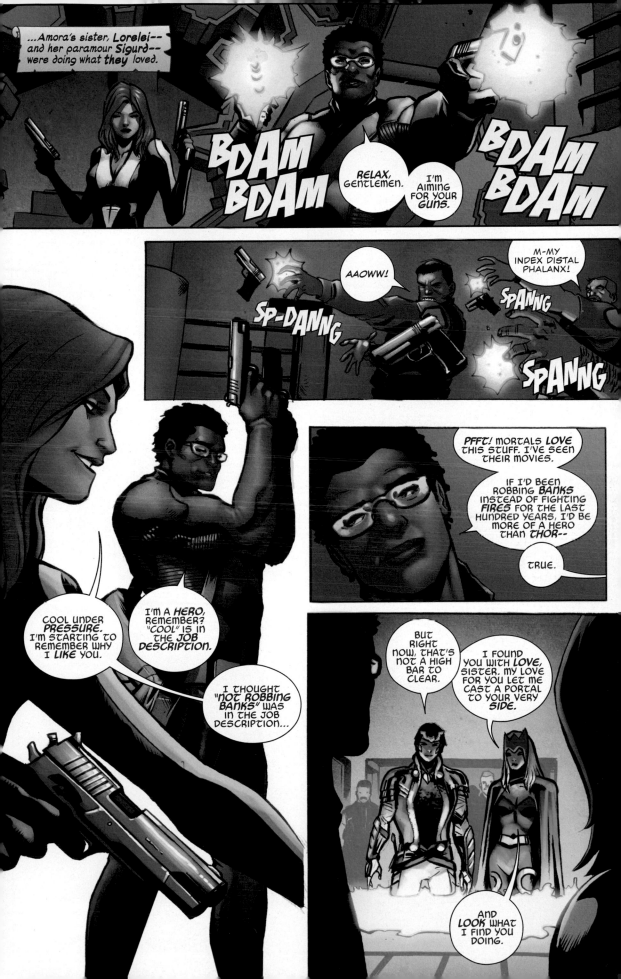

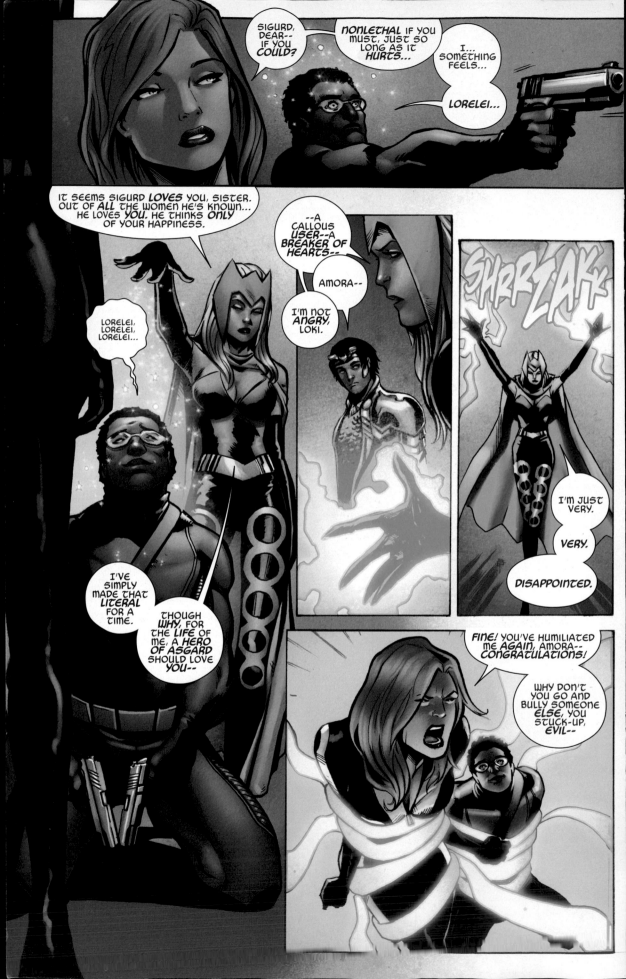

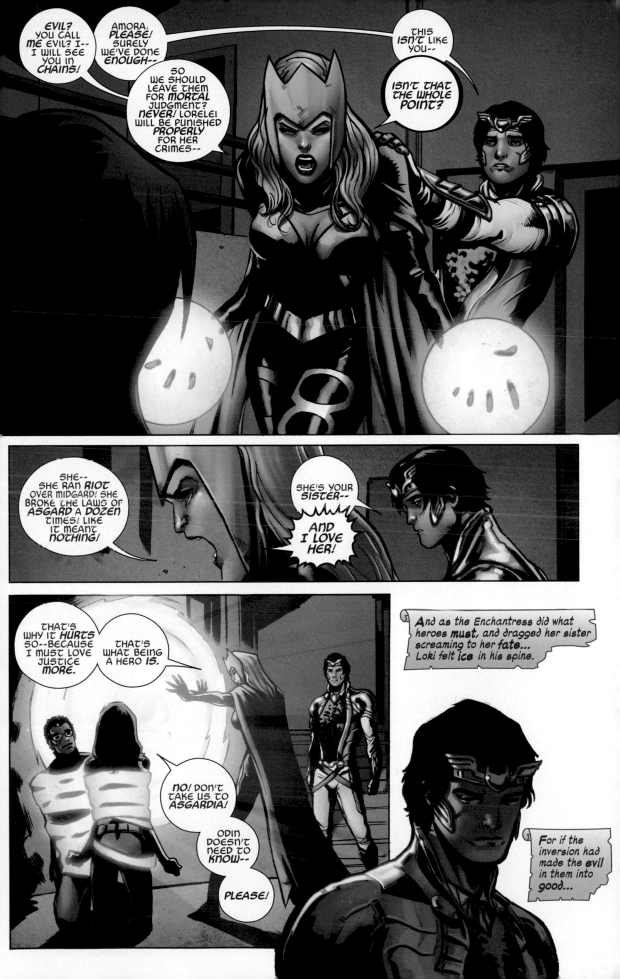

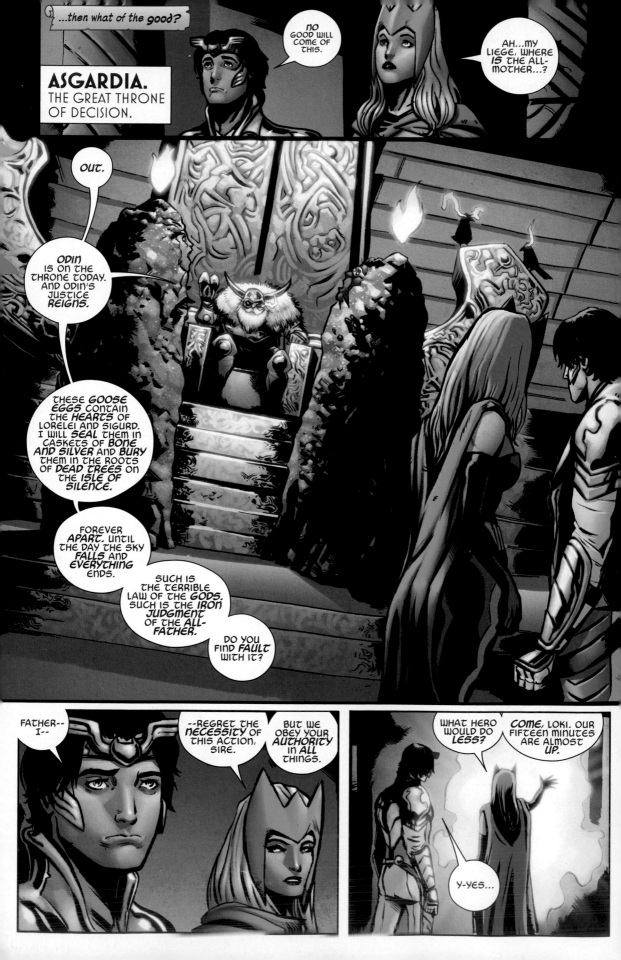

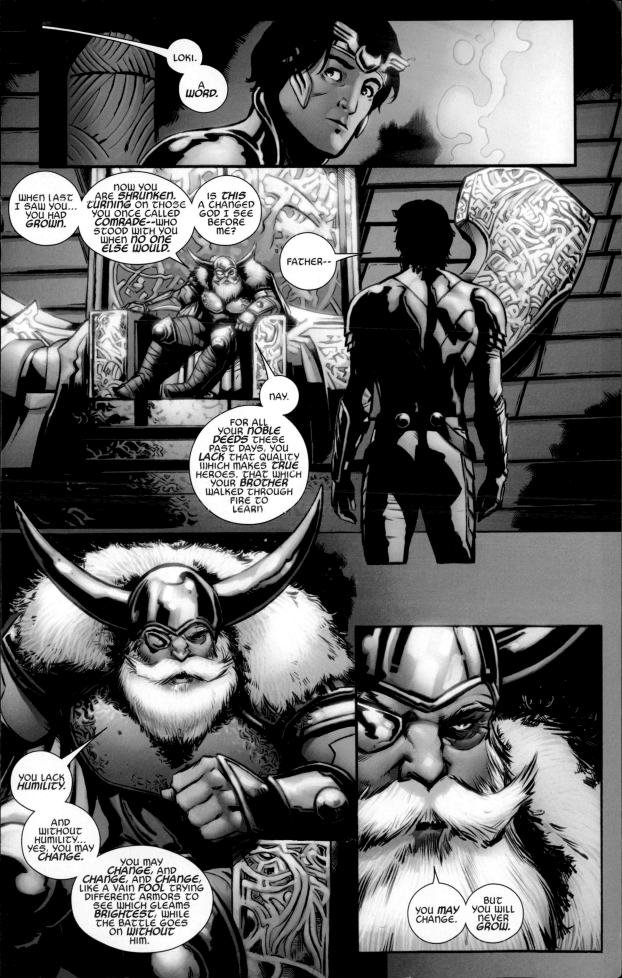

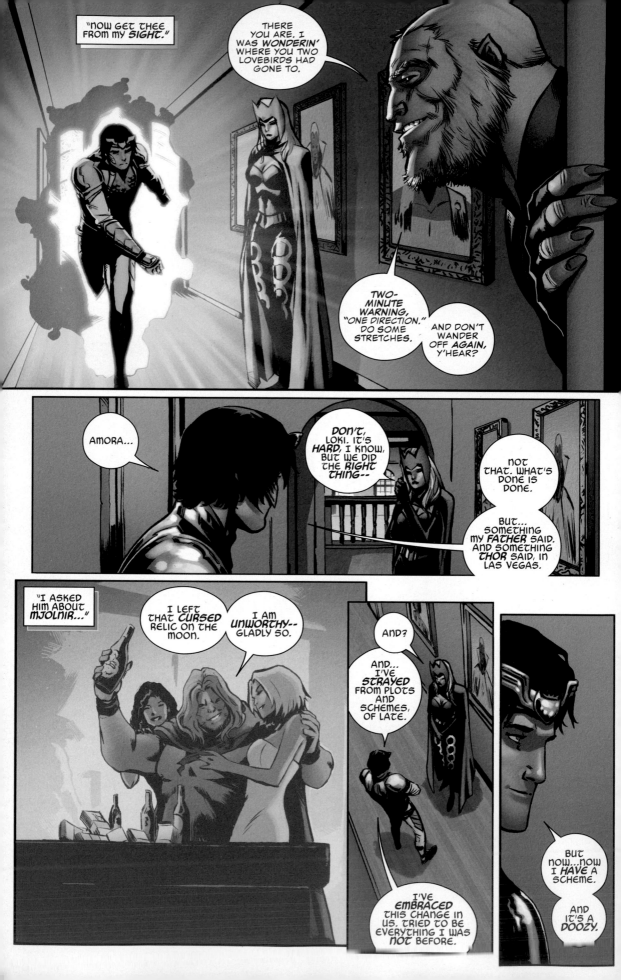

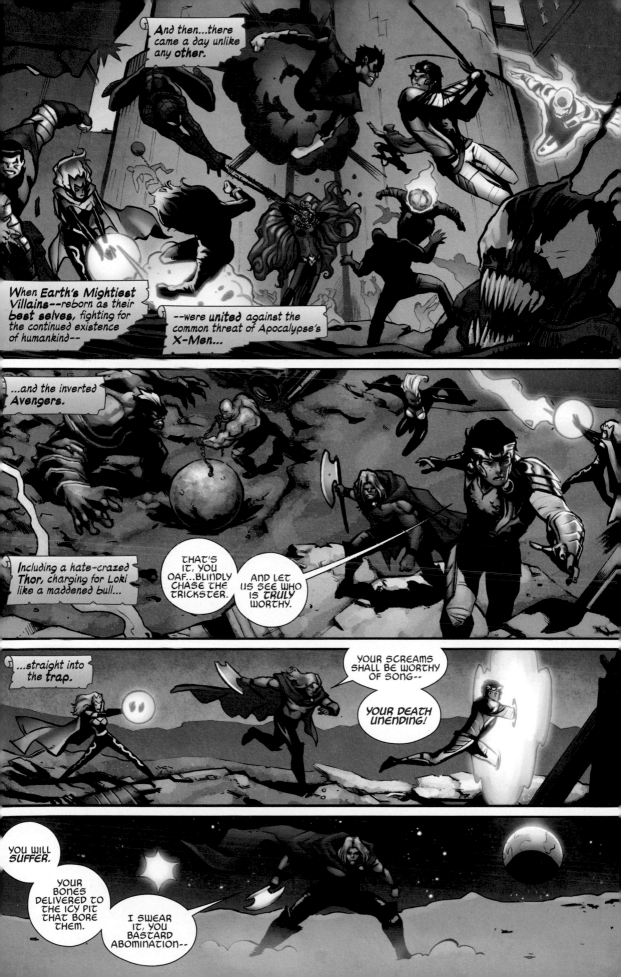

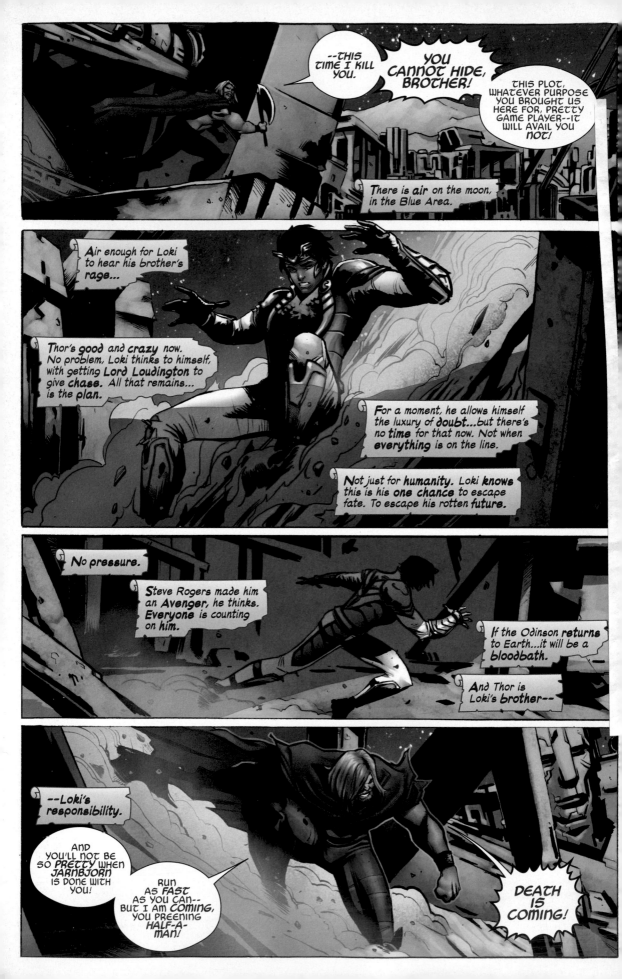

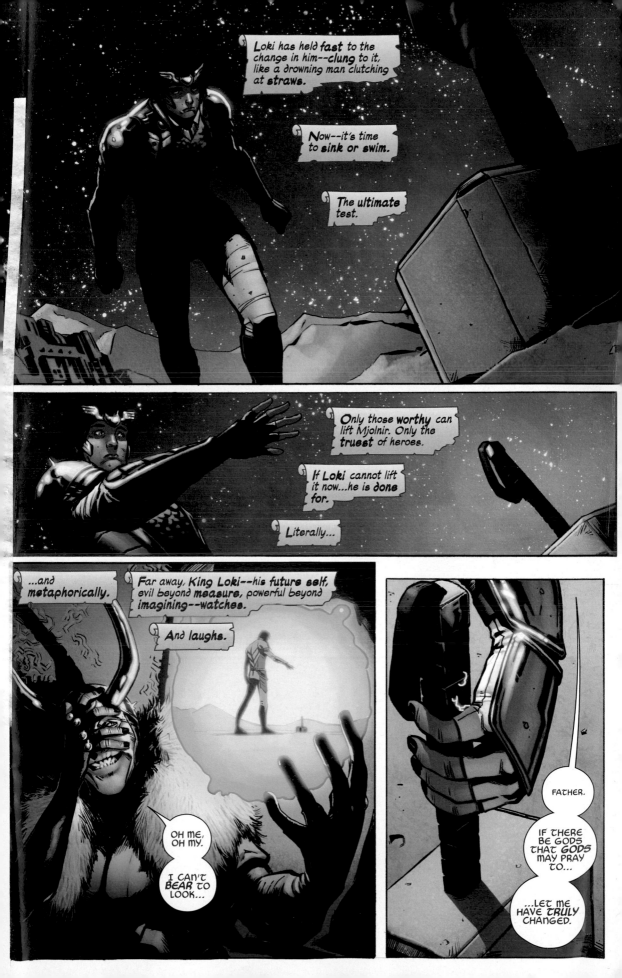

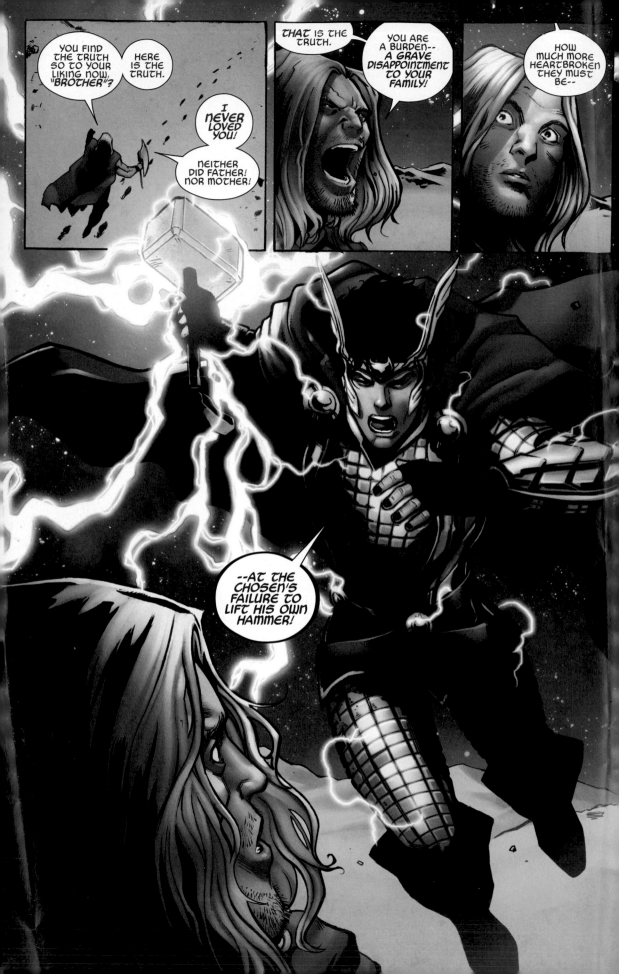

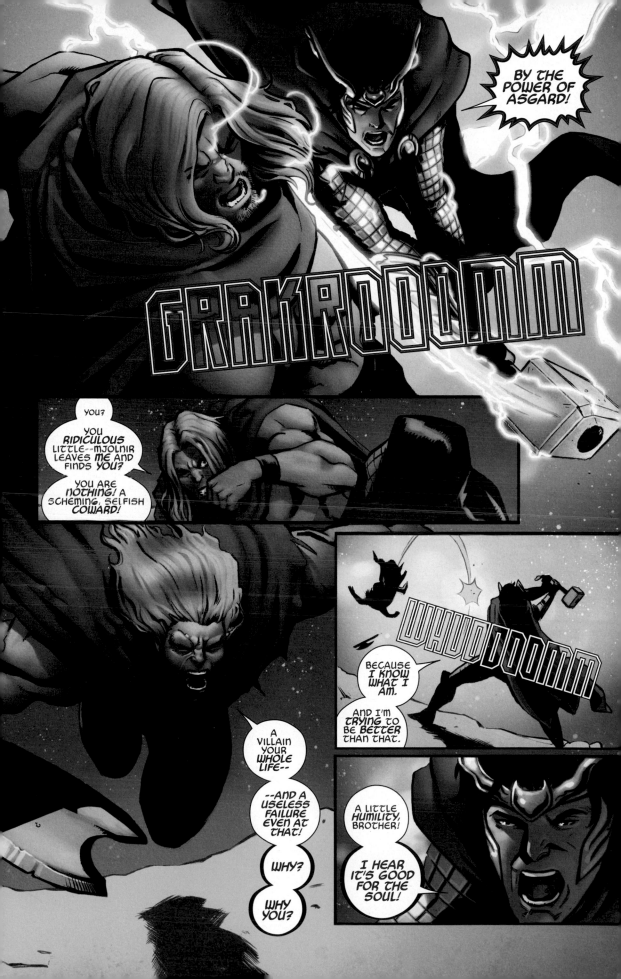

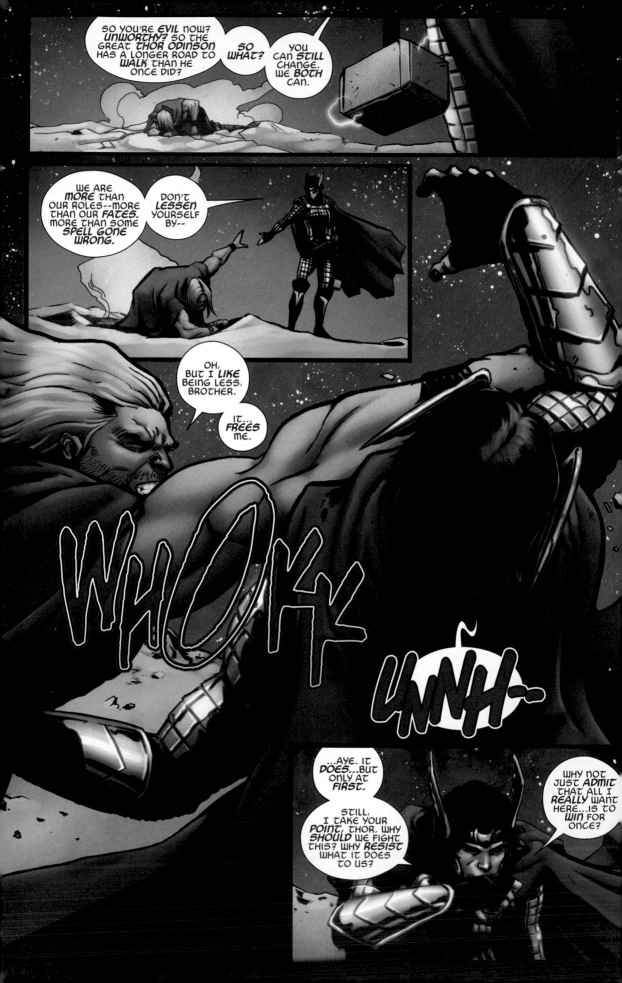

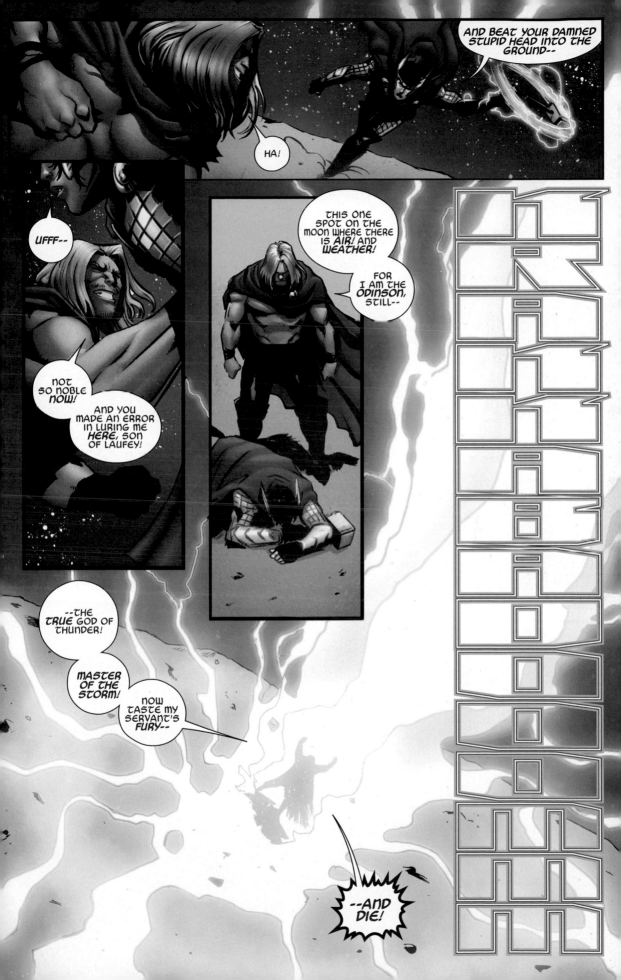

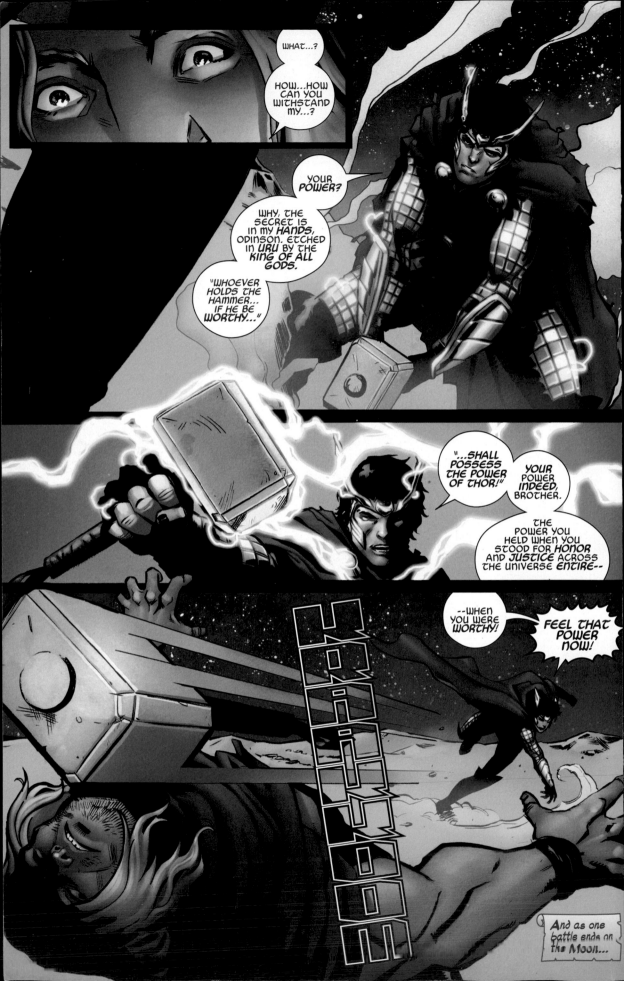

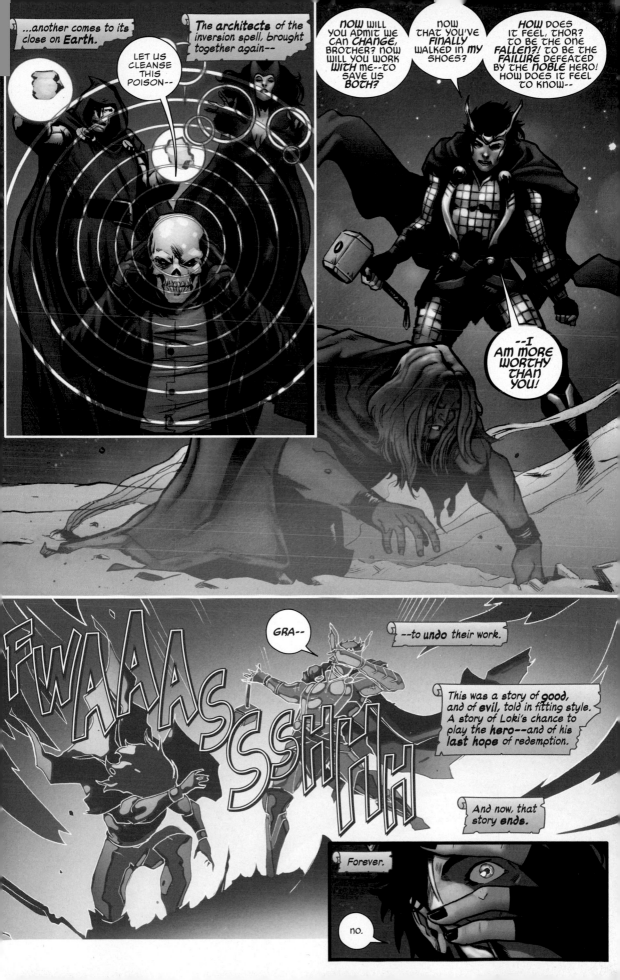

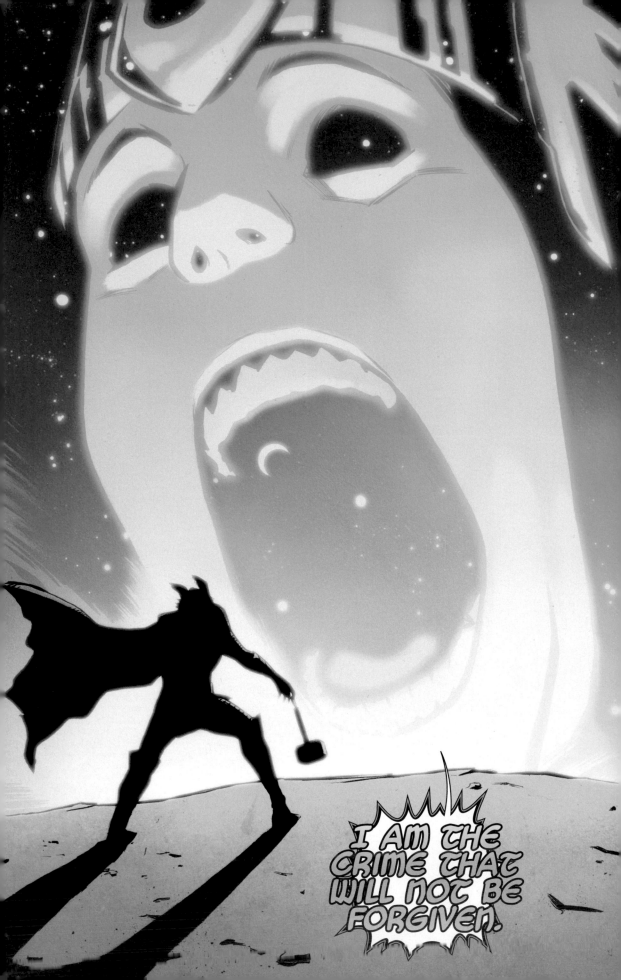

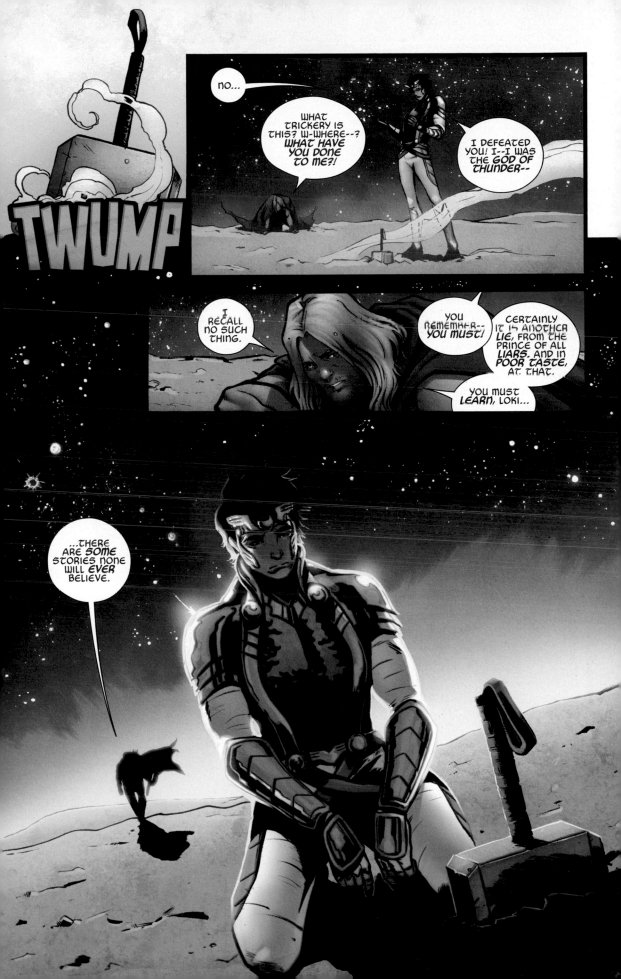

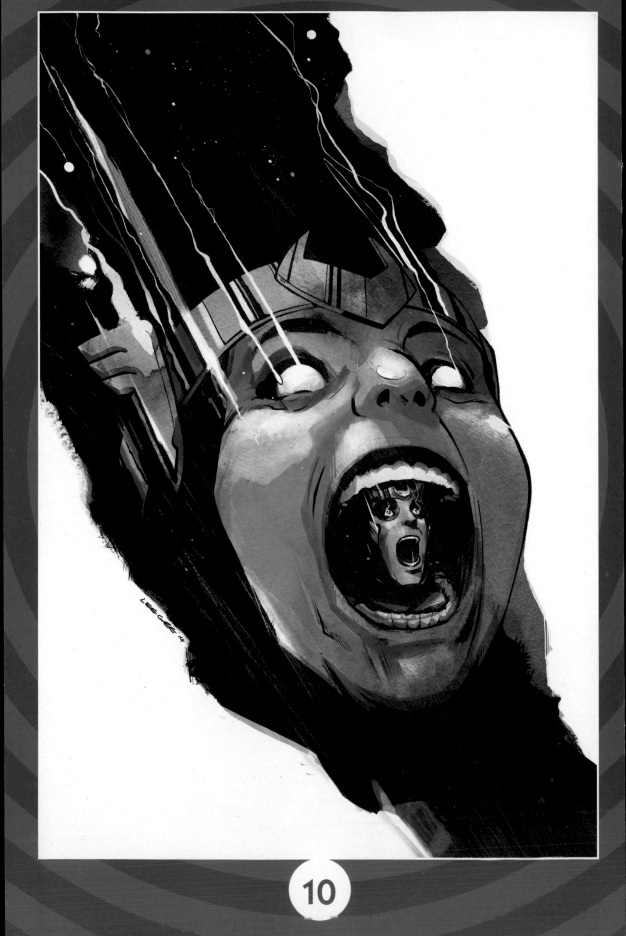

10

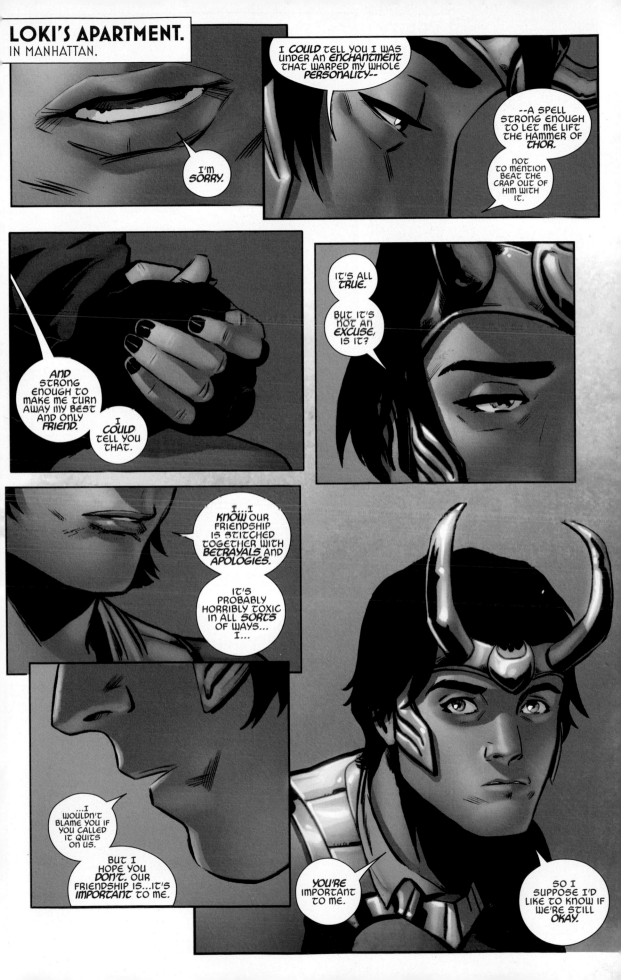

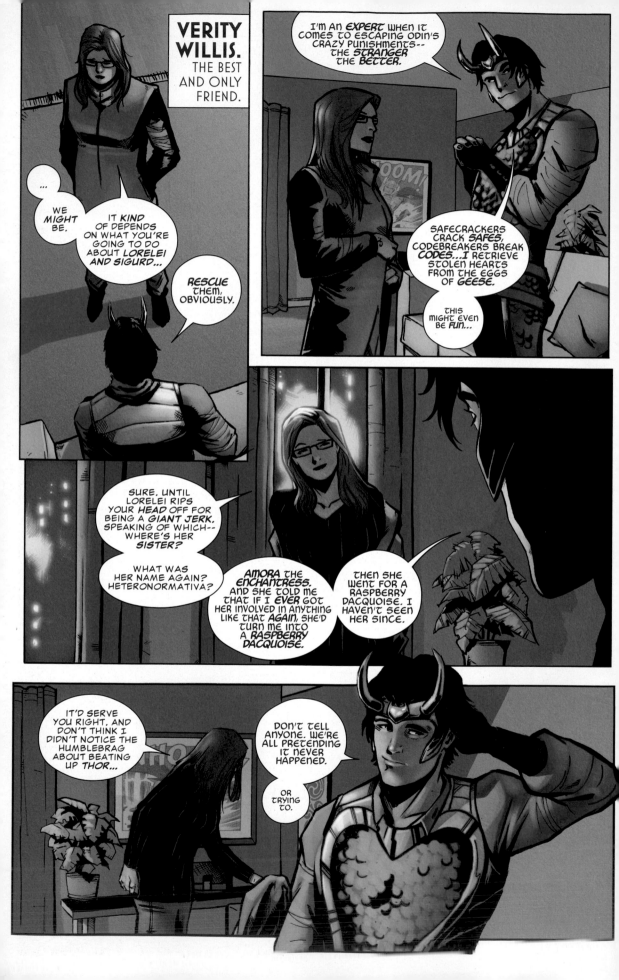

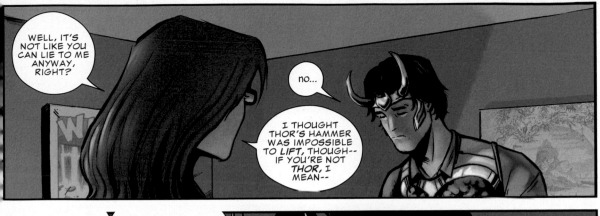

WELL, IT'S NOT LIKE YOU CAN LIE TO ME ANYWAY, RIGHT?

no...

I THOUGHT THOR'S HAMMER WAS IMPOSSIBLE TO *LIFT*, THOUGH-- IF YOU'RE NOT *THOR*, I MEAN--

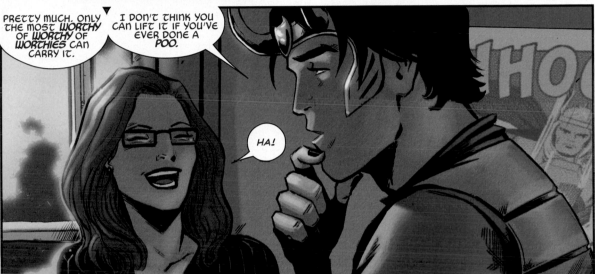

PRETTY MUCH. ONLY THE MOST *WORTHY* OF *WORTHY* OF *WORTHIES* CAN CARRY IT.

I DON'T THINK YOU CAN LIFT IT IF YOU'VE EVER DONE A *POO*.

HA!

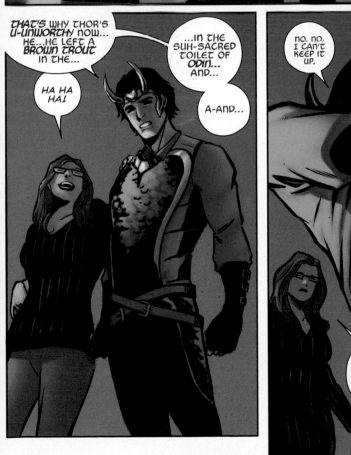

THAT'S WHY THOR'S U-*UNWORTHY* NOW... HE...HE LEFT A *BROWN TROUT* IN THE...

...IN THE SUH-SACRED TOILET OF *ODIN*... AND...

A-AND...

HA HA HA!

NO. NO, I CAN'T KEEP IT UP.

I'M *JOKING*, VERITY. *NONE* OF THAT REALLY HAPPENED.

NO *KIDDING*, LOKI, YOU DON'T HAVE TO *EXPLAIN* IT--

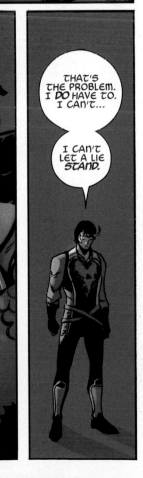

THAT'S THE PROBLEM. I *DO* HAVE TO. I CAN'T...

I CAN'T LET A LIE *STAND*.

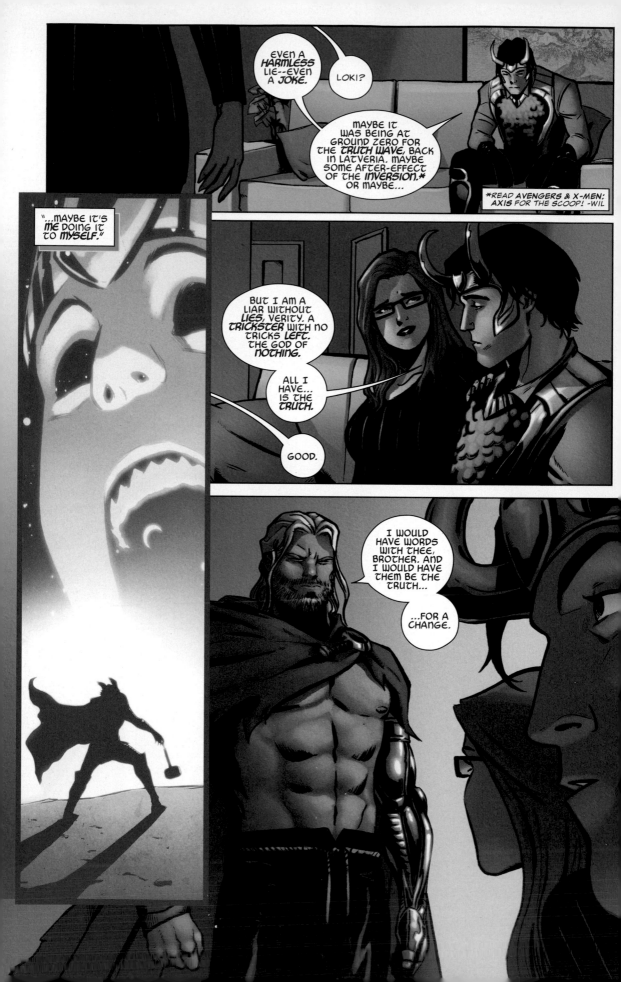

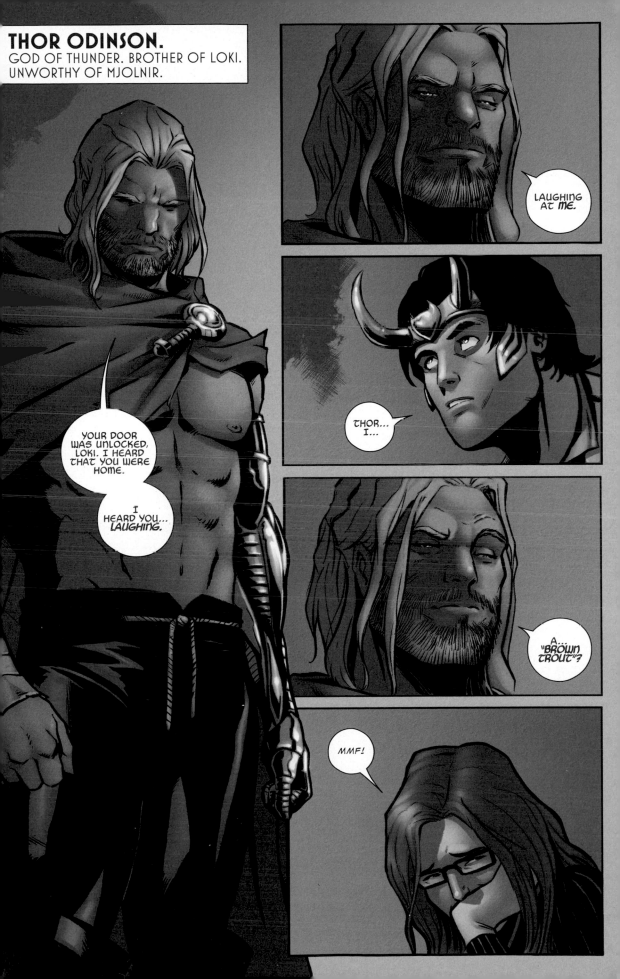

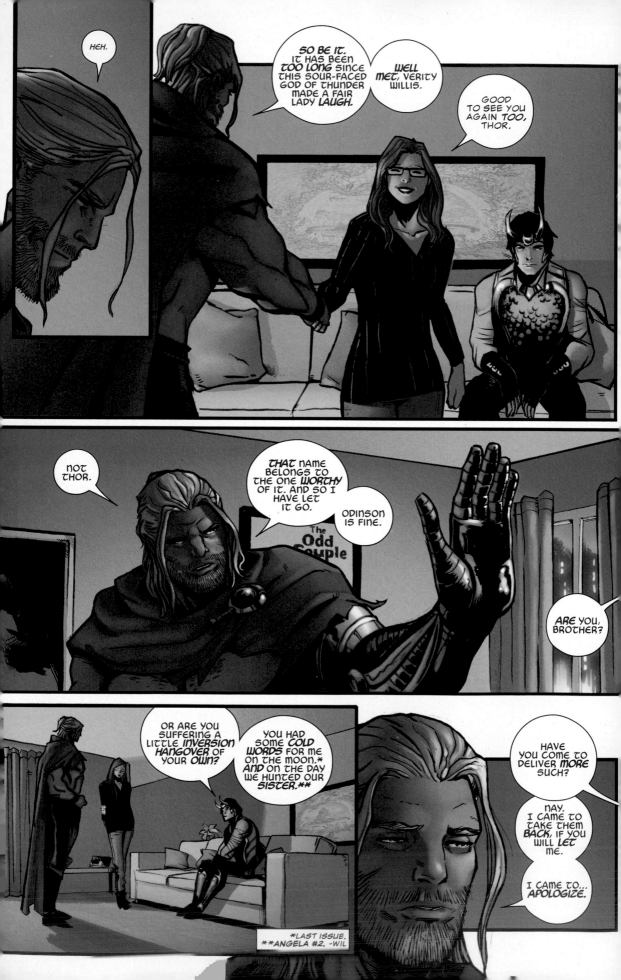

*LAST ISSUE.
**ANGELA #2. -WIL

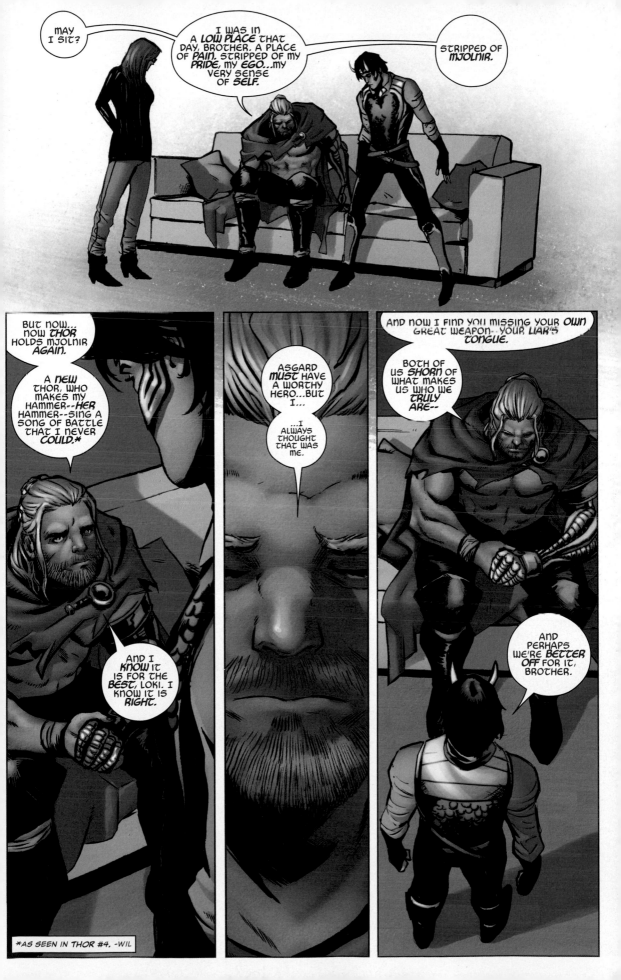

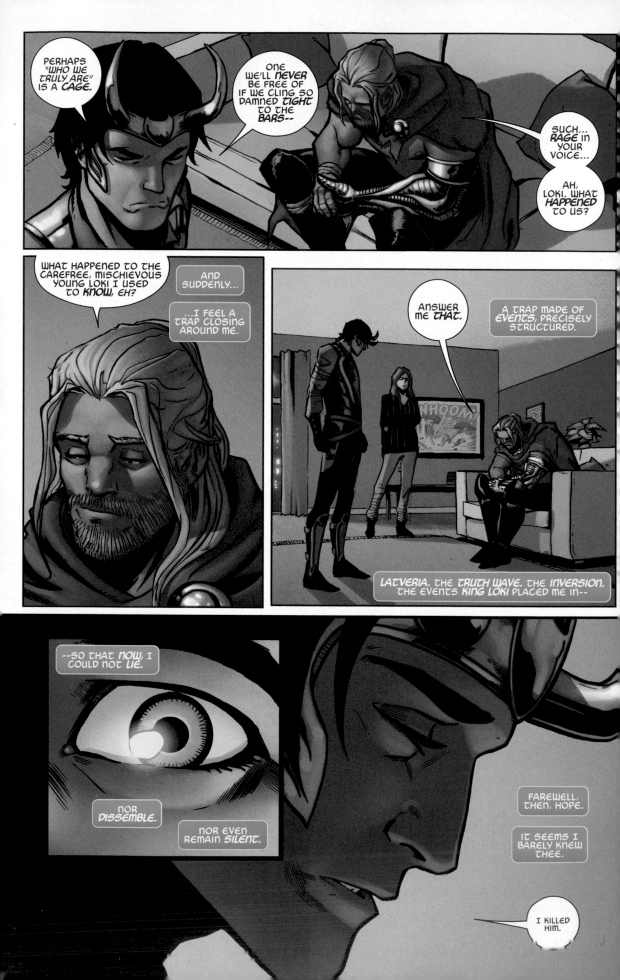

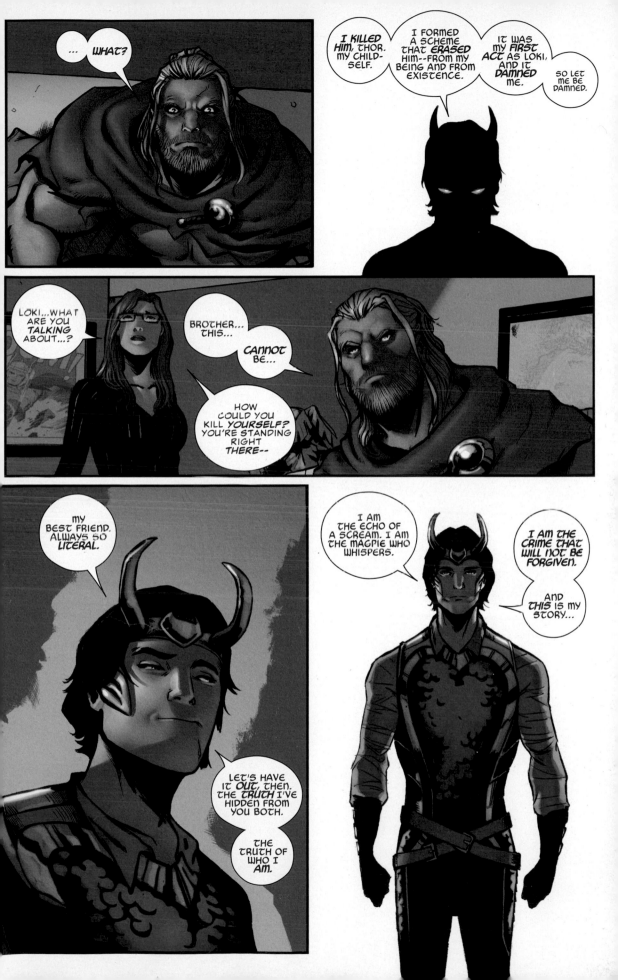

THIS IS THE STORY OF LOKI.

LOKI, WHO WAS DOOMED TO NEVER BE ANYTHING BUT LOKI — LOKI THE BAD SON, LOKI THE VILLAIN — UNTIL THE DAY HE DIED.

SO...HE DIED.

WHICH WAS, OF COURSE, HIS GREATEST SCHEME OF ALL.

FOR SOON HE WAS REBORN INTO A NEW, YOUTHFUL BODY, FREE TO CHOOSE HIS OWN FATE. "KID LOKI" — A NEW PERSONALITY, FREE FROM THE TAINT OF THE OLD...AT FIRST. FOR THIS NEW LOKI TOOK THE FADING ECHO OF THE OLD – BOTH GHOST AND COPY — TO ADVISE HIM AND GIVE HIM KNOWLEDGE.

ALL LOKIS, IT SEEMS, MUST DAMN THEMSELVES EARLY.

THE GHOST-COPY, CALLED IKOL, HAD NEITHER POWER NOR MAGIC. BUT WHAT HE HAD WAS ENOUGH – KID LOKI'S EAR. WITH THIS, HE CRAFTED A SCHEME THAT WOULD GIVE HIM CONTROL OF THE GODLING'S BODY...

...AND CAST KID LOKI'S VERY SELF – HIS MIND AND SOUL AND BEING — INTO TOTAL ANNIHILATION, DESTROYING THE CHILD FOREVER.

PERHAPS ALL LOKIS MUST FALL TO THE VOID, AS WELL.

AFTER THE DEED WAS DONE, IKOL-LOKI — THE THIRD LOKI – FOUND HIMSELF TRAPPED IN THE SHAPE OF HIS VICTIM, PLAYING THE ROLE OF THE GOOD TRICKSTER DESPITE HIS WORST INTENTIONS. AND THOUGH HE CHANGED THAT SHAPE — AGING TO YOUNG-MANHOOD — HE WAS STILL TORMENTED BY SHAME AND GUILT AND SELF-LOATHING. BY THE ECHO OF A FINAL SCREAM — KID LOKI'S ACCUSATION THAT HE COULD NEVER TRULY CHANGE.

SO HE TRIED TO BE BETTER. HE TRIED TO CHANGE. HE TRIED TO GROW. AND TO THIS END, HE MADE A DEAL WITH THE ALL-MOTHER, TO PERFORM MISSIONS FOR ASGARD TO ERASE HIS EVIL PAST. AND SO WAS BORN...

...THE AGENT OF ASGARD.

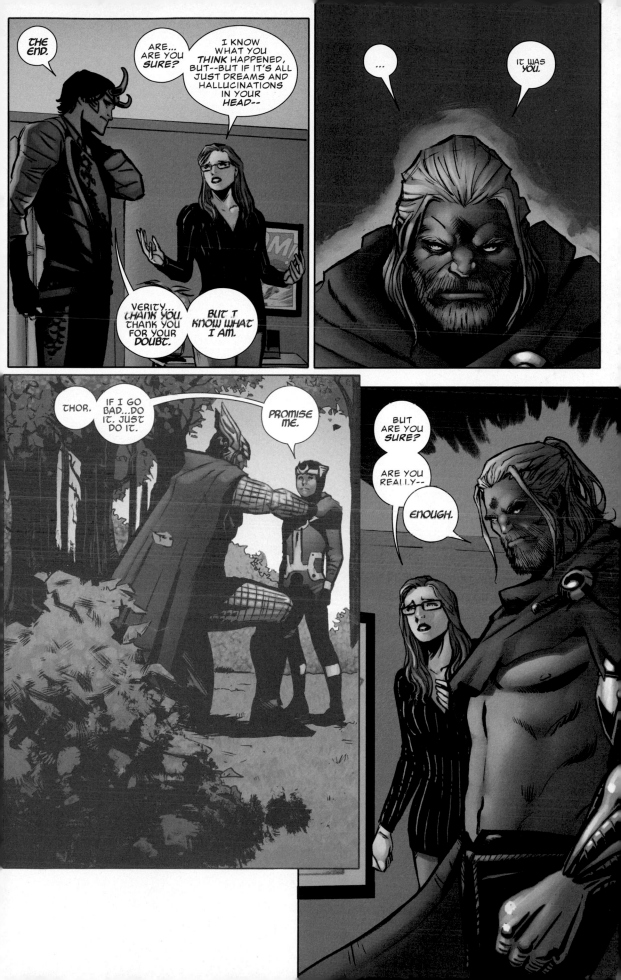

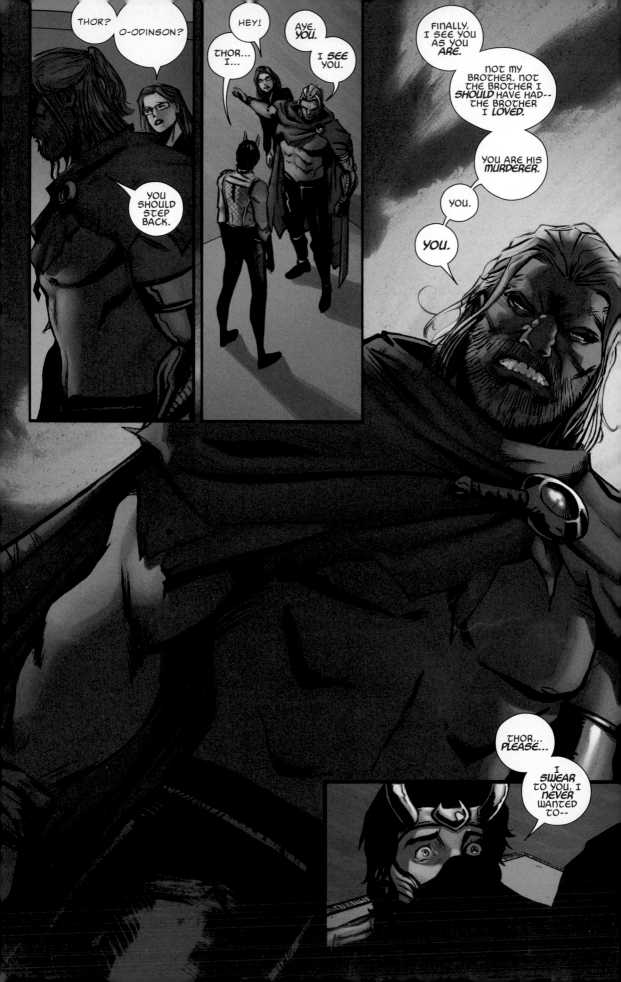

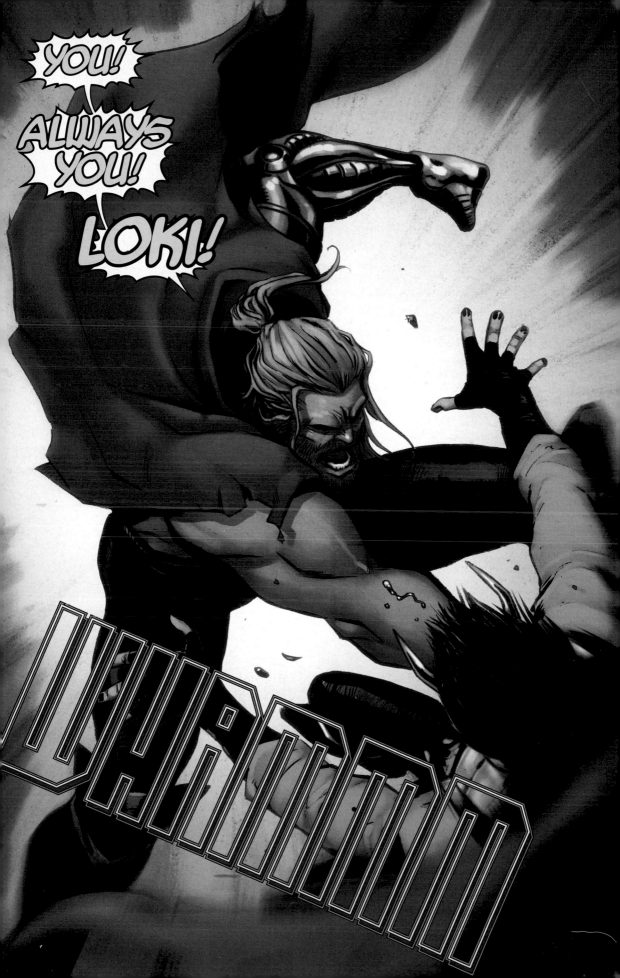

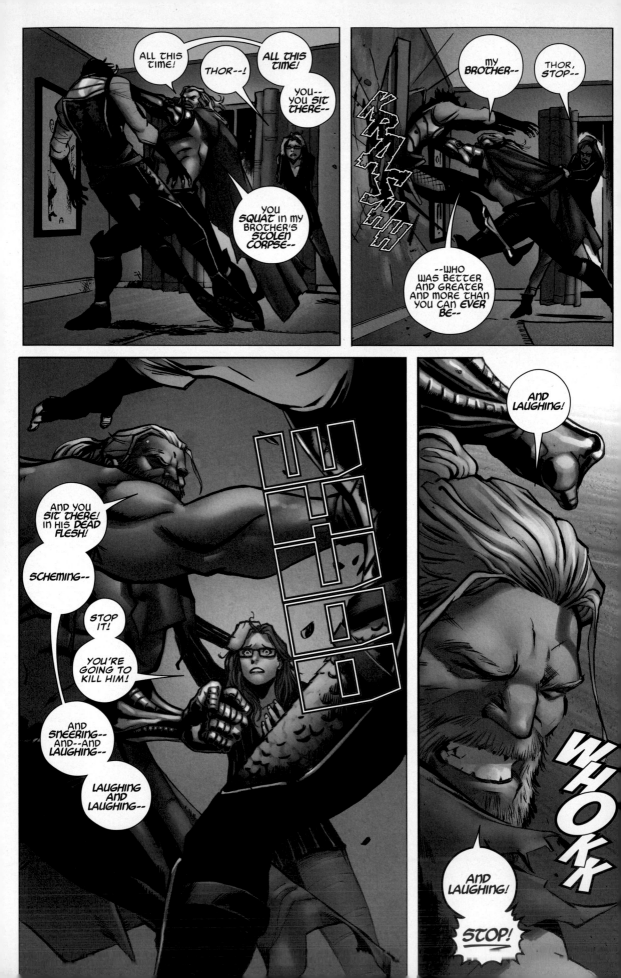

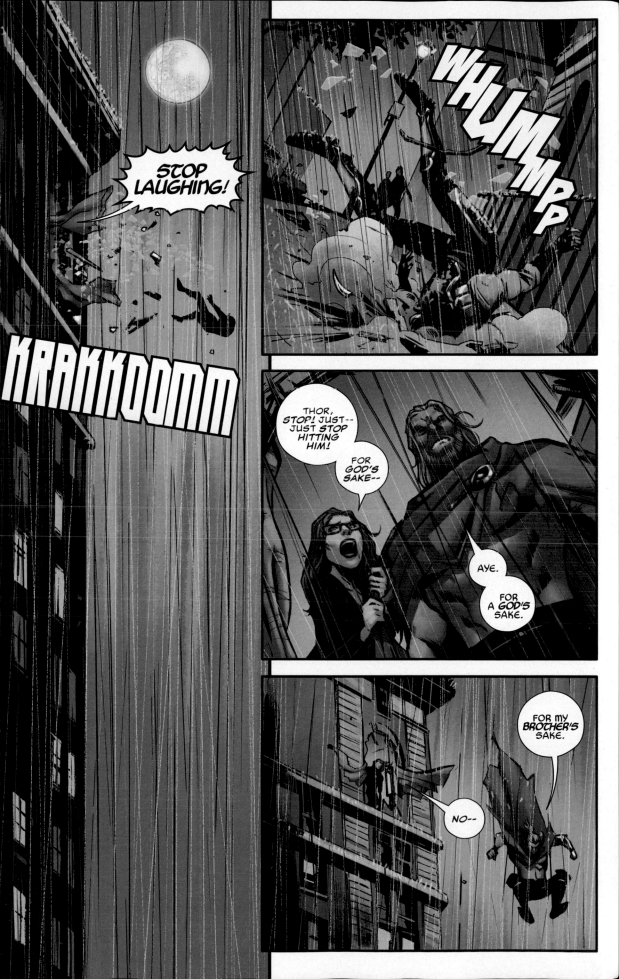

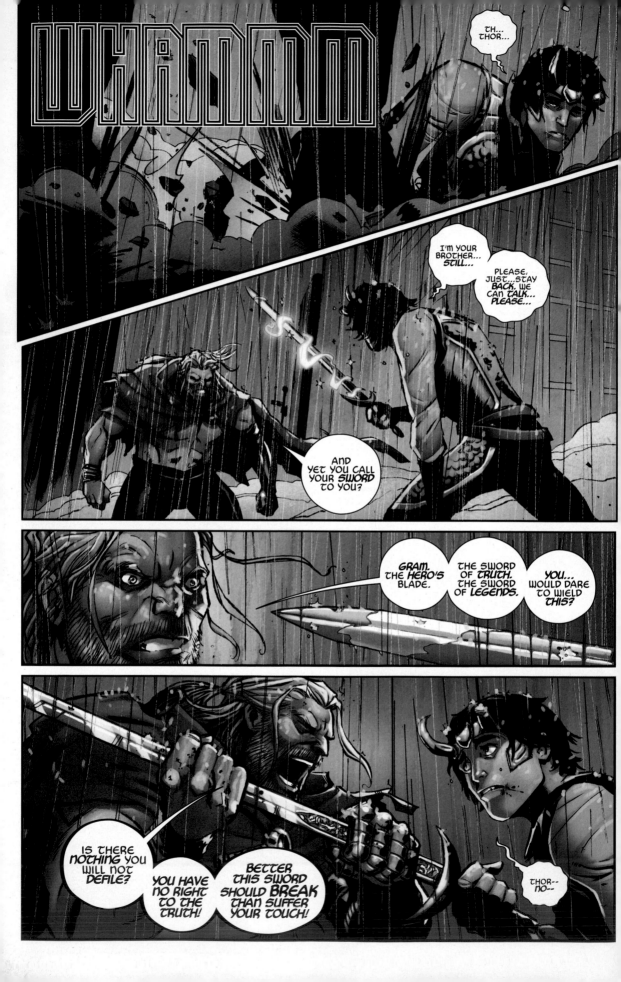

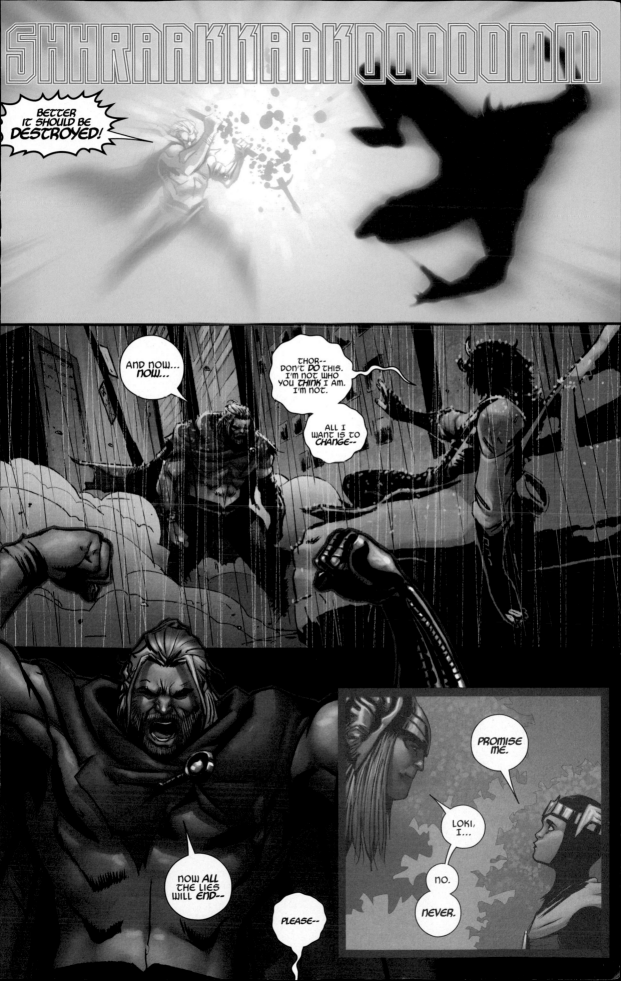

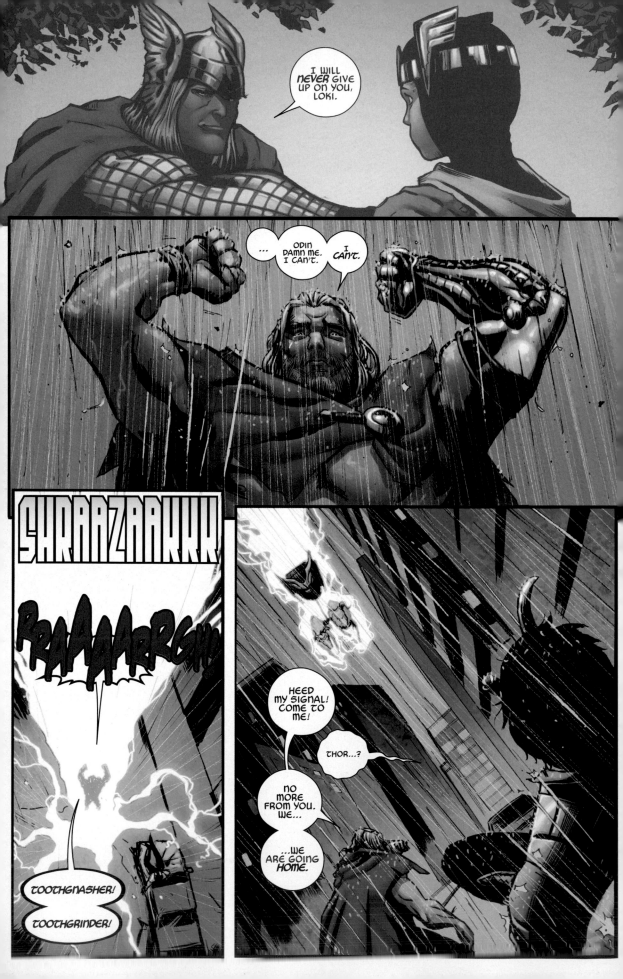

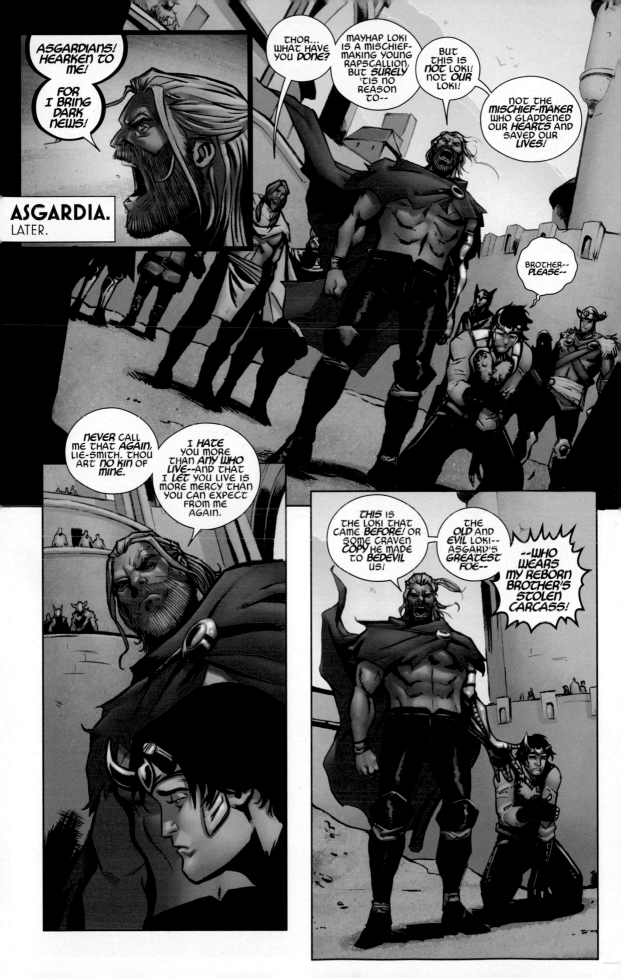

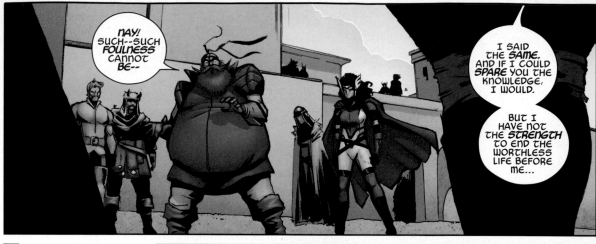

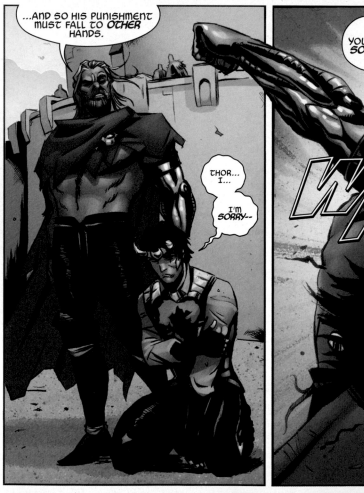

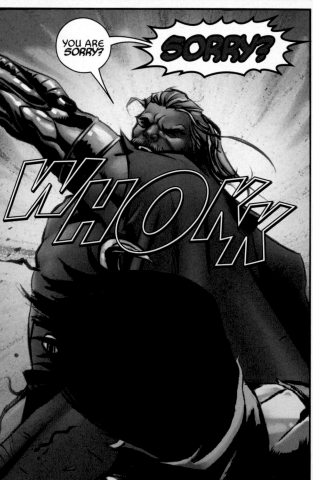

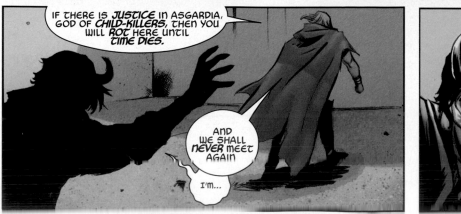

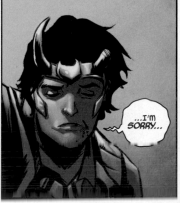

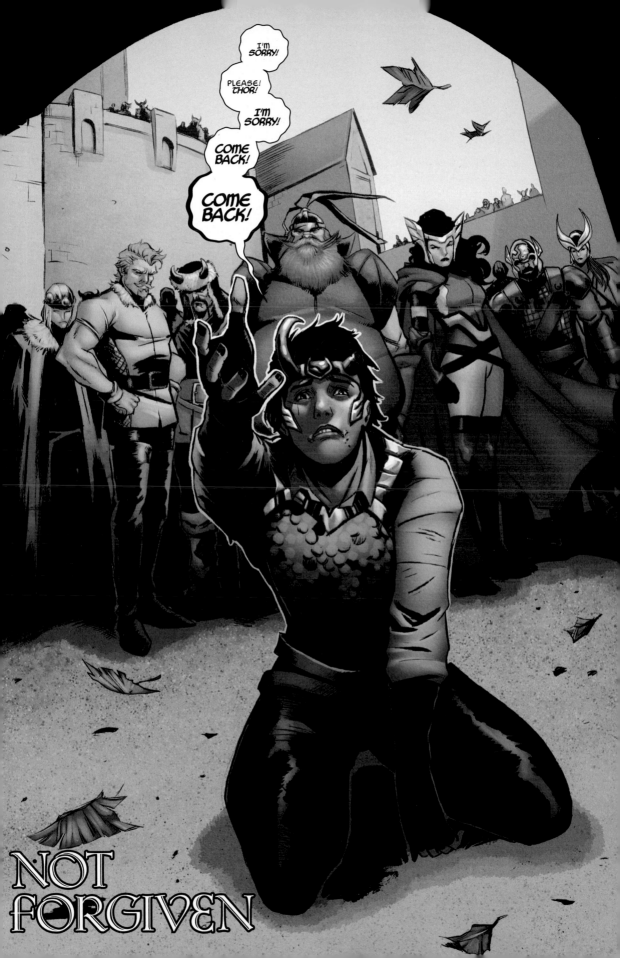

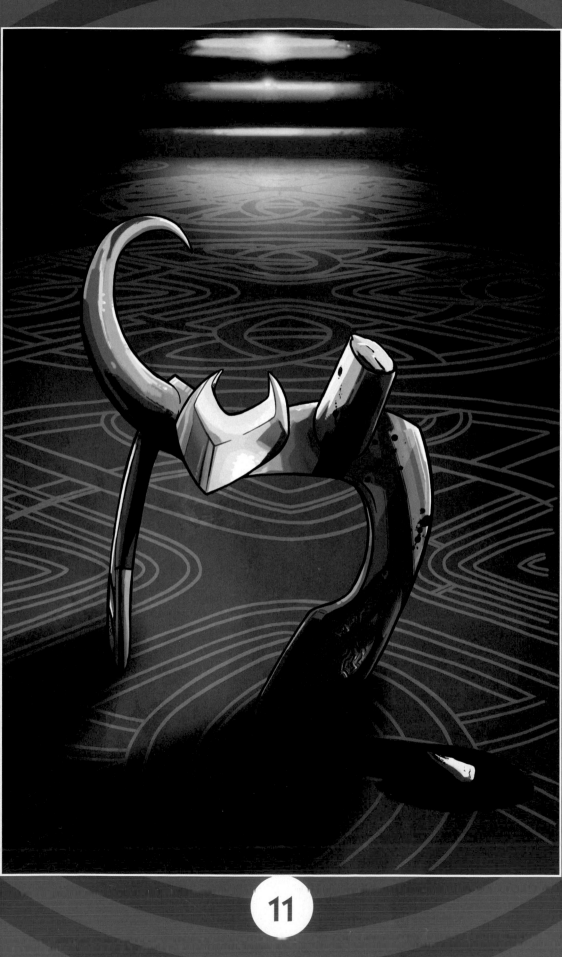

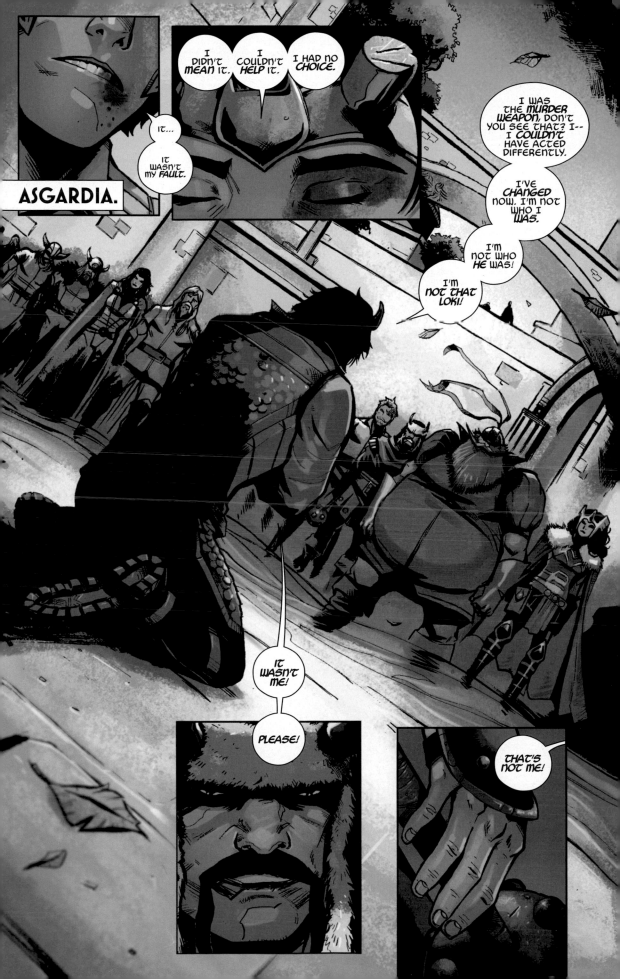

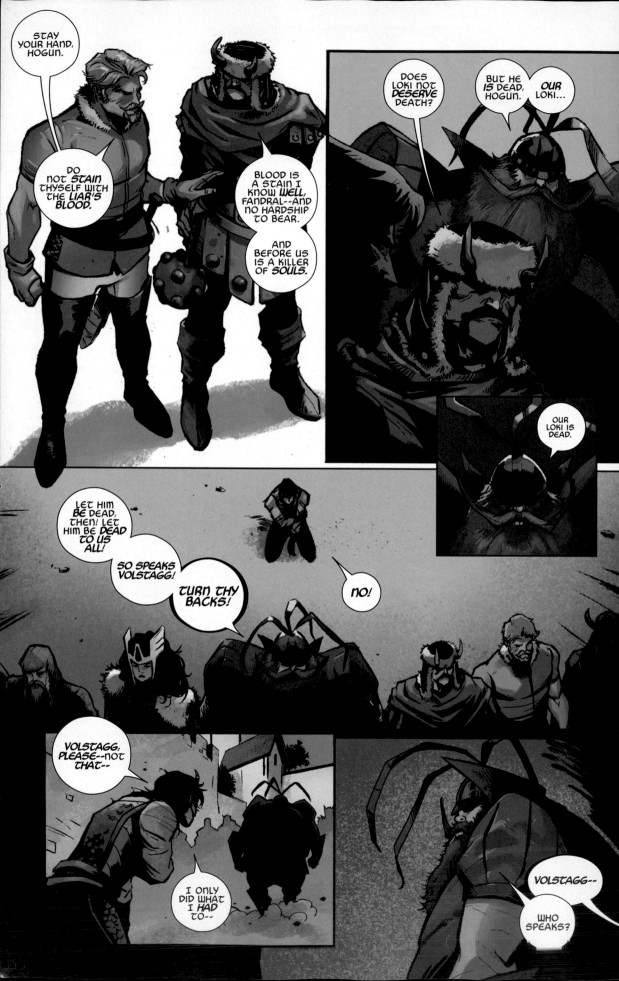

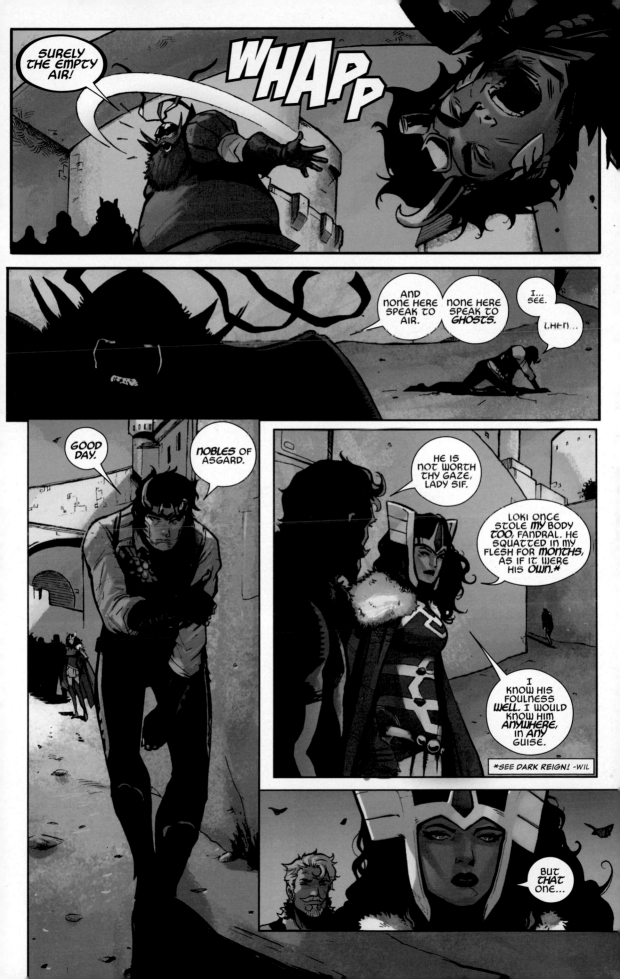

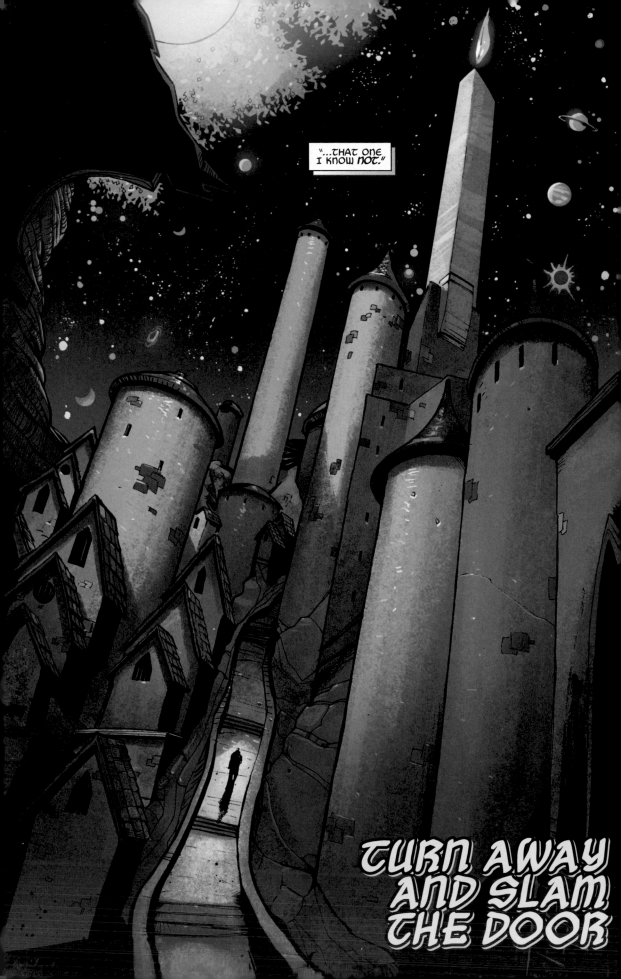

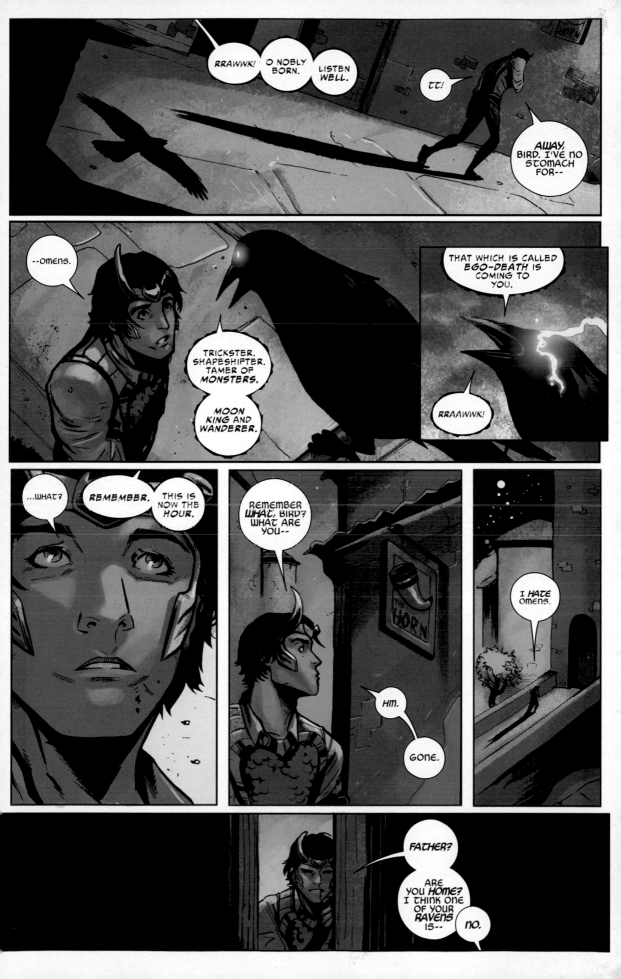

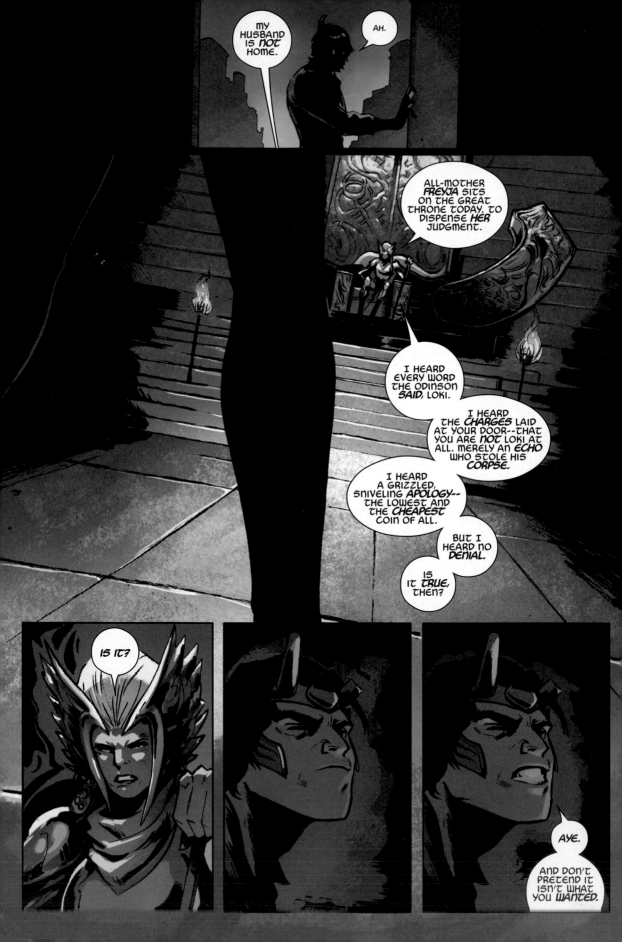

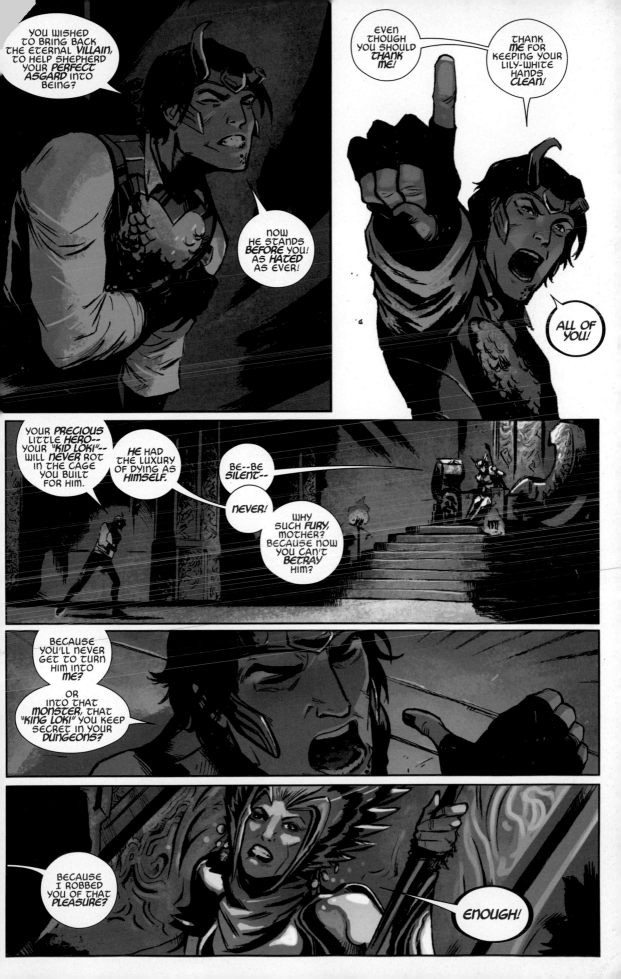

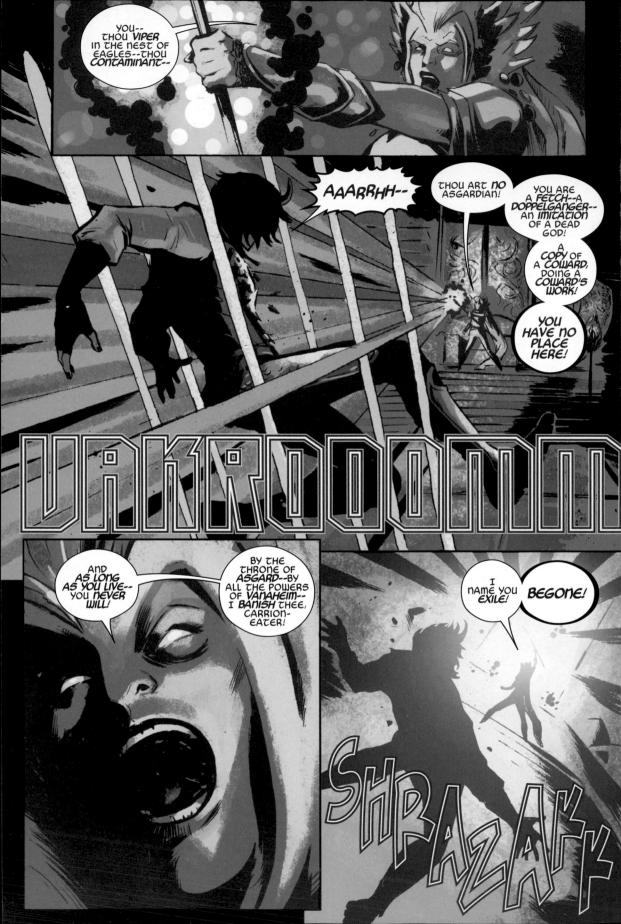

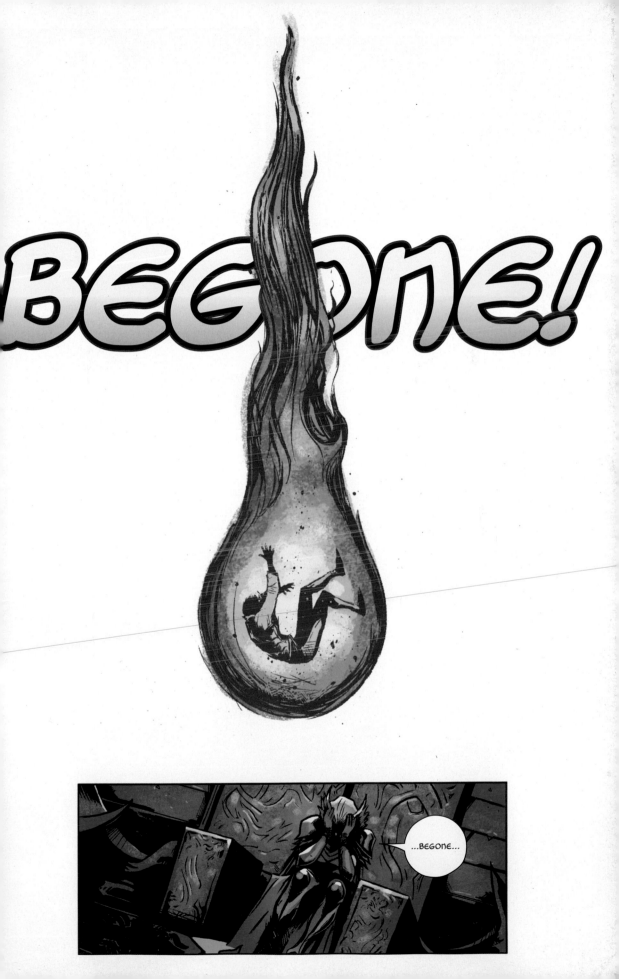

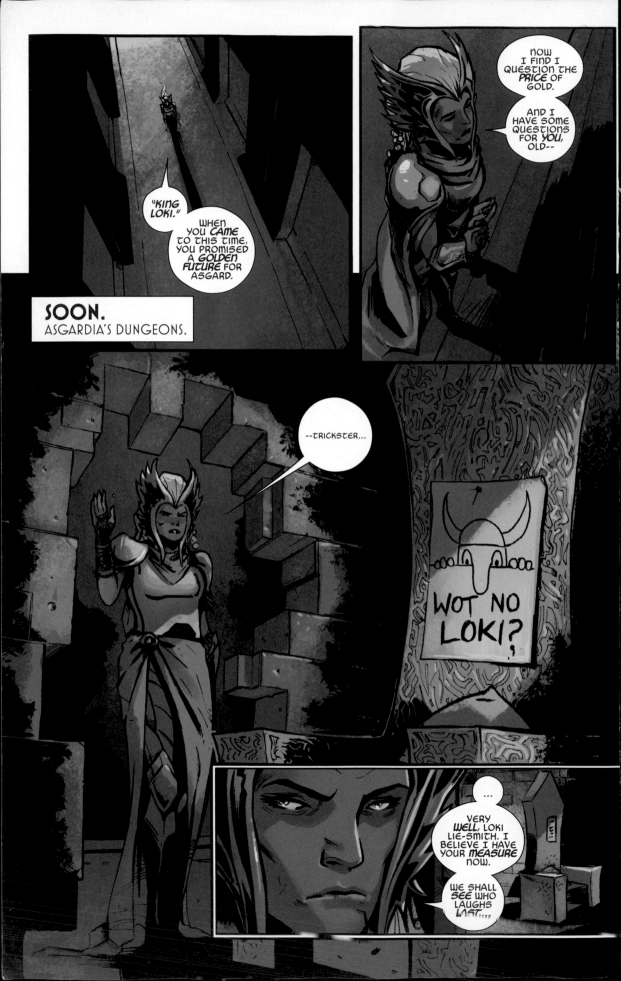

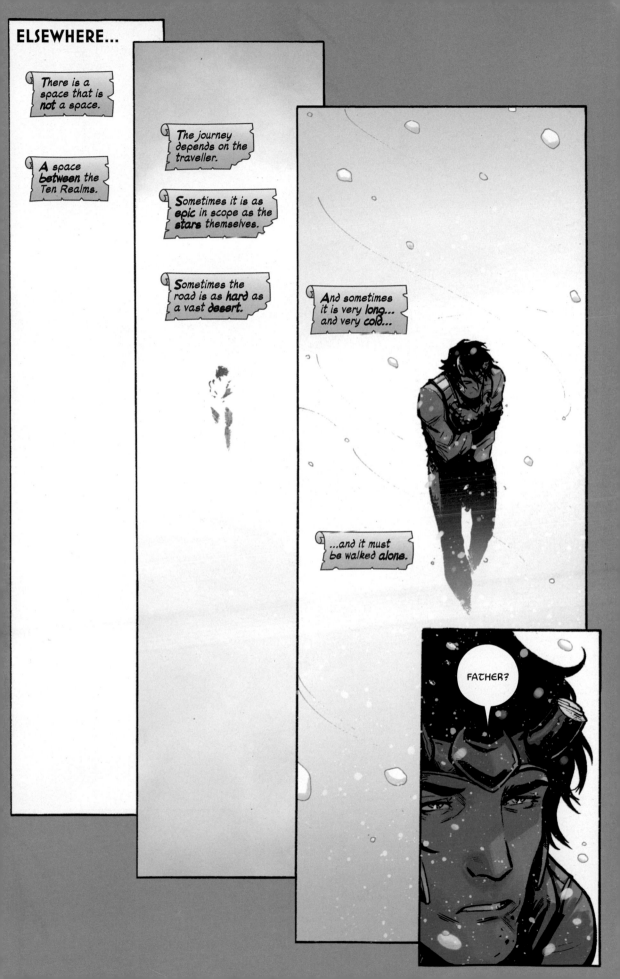

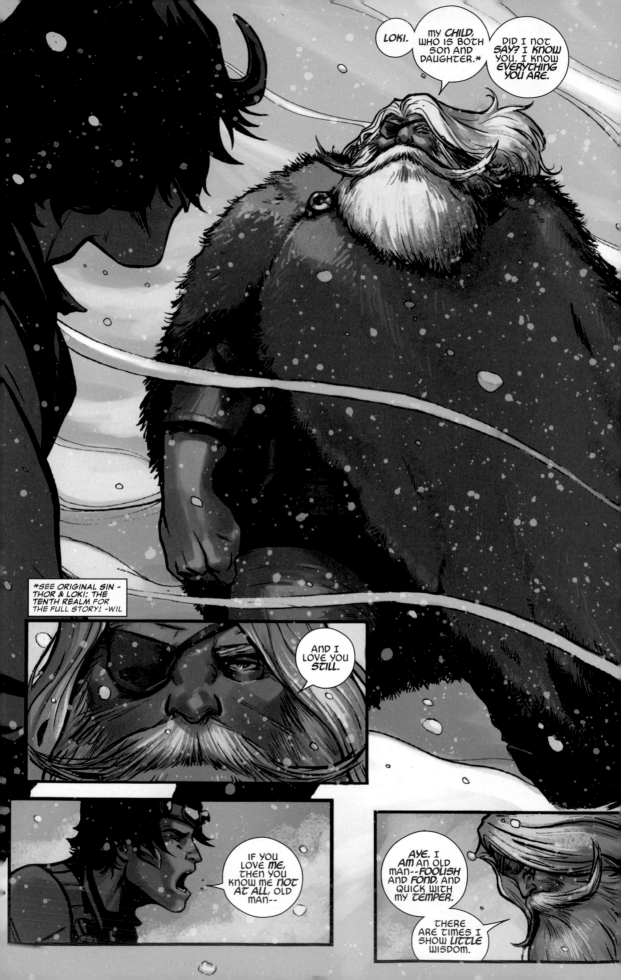

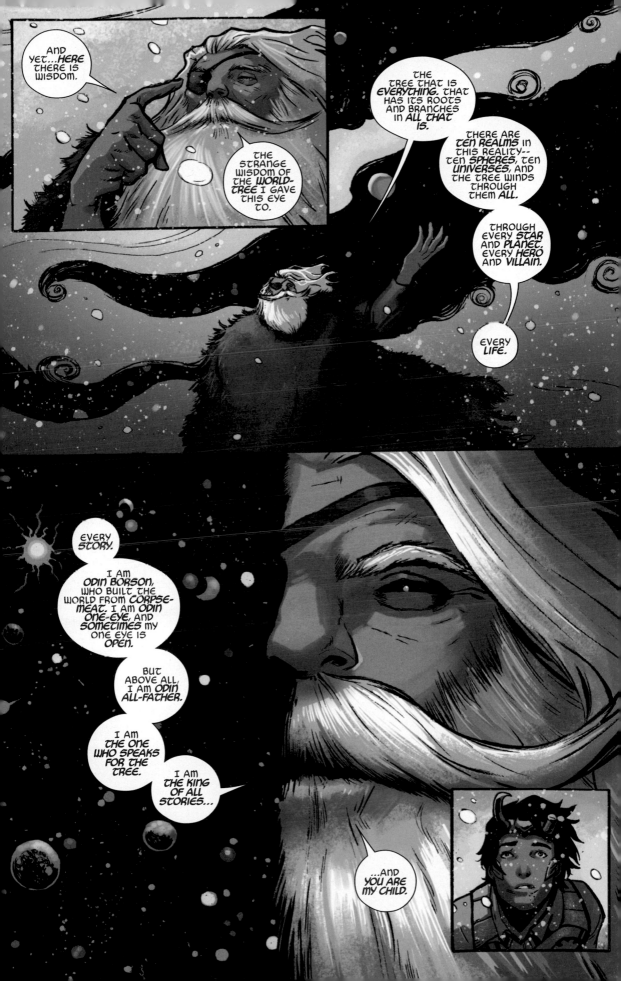

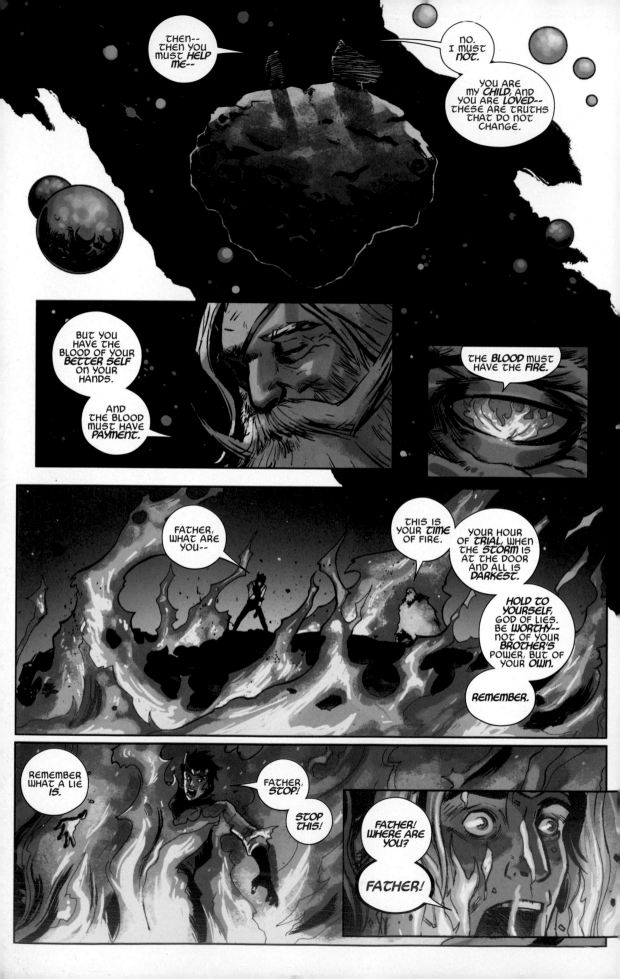

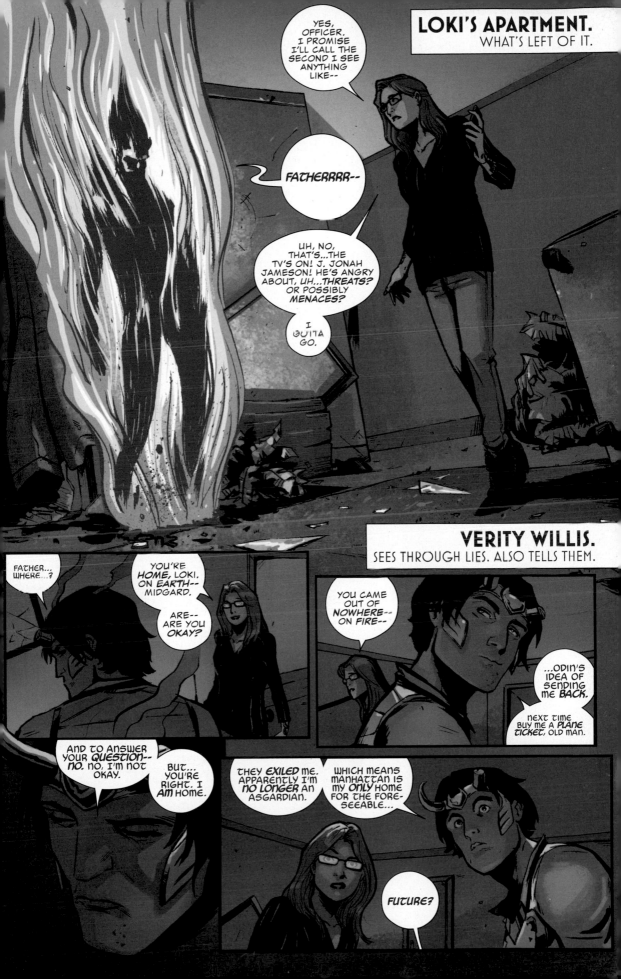

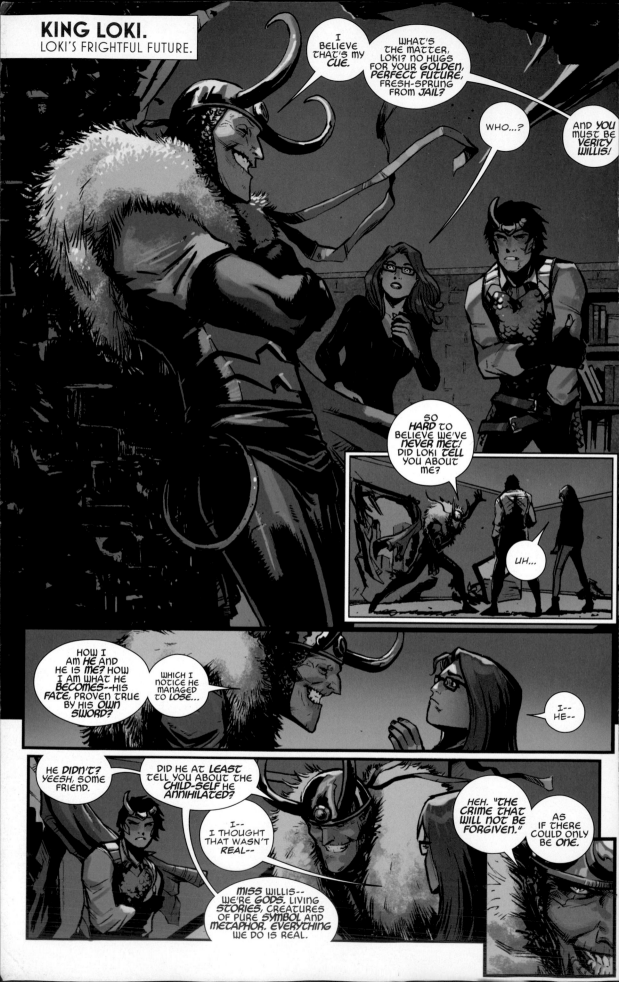

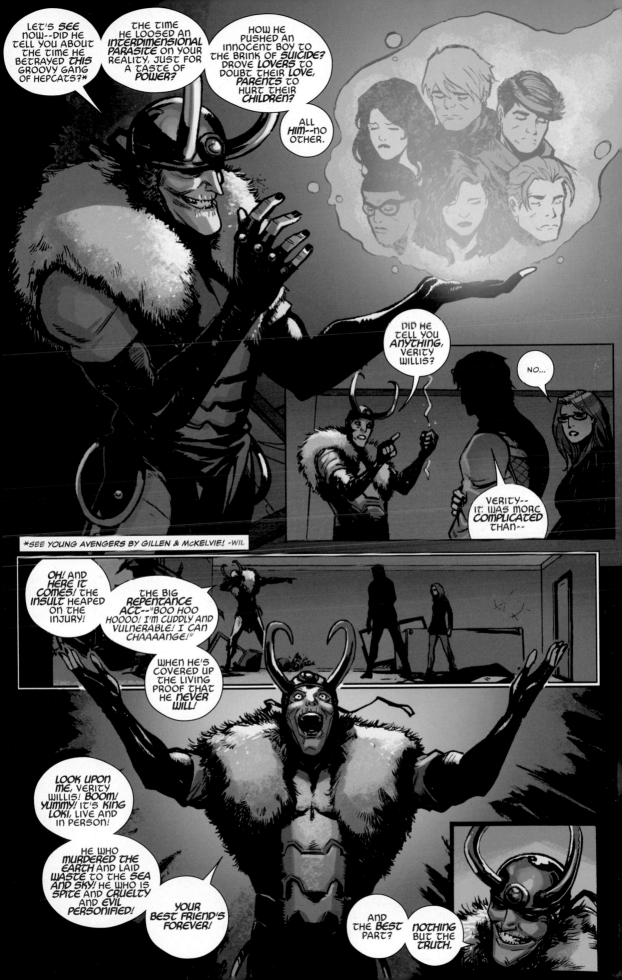

*SEE YOUNG AVENGERS BY GILLEN & McKELVIE! -WIL

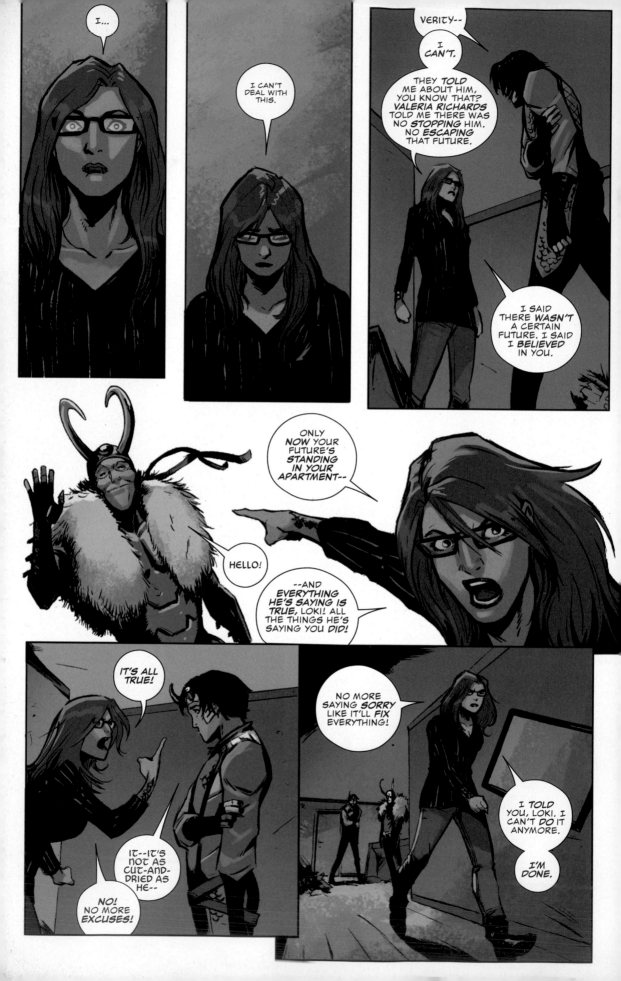

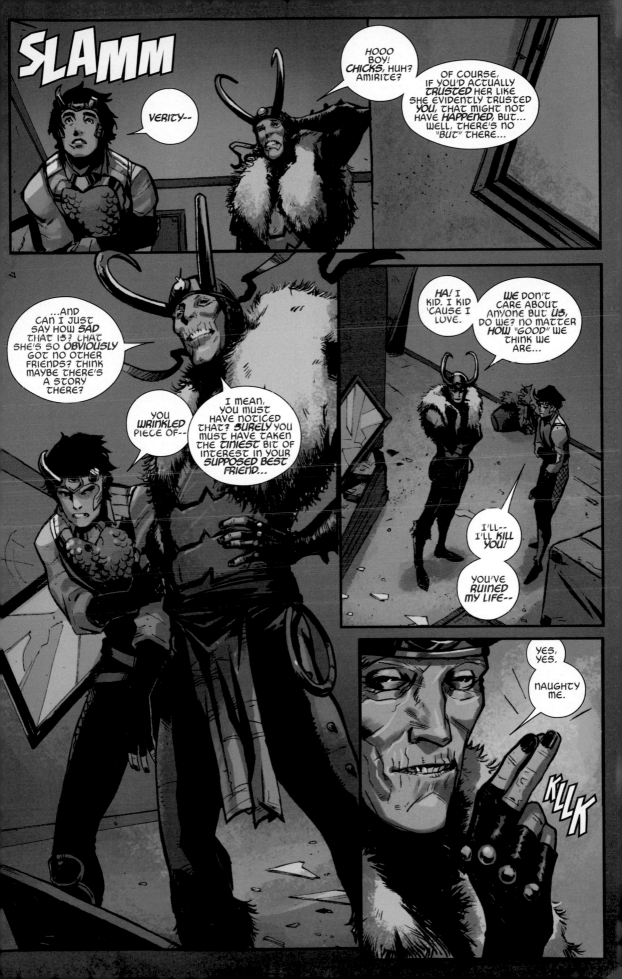

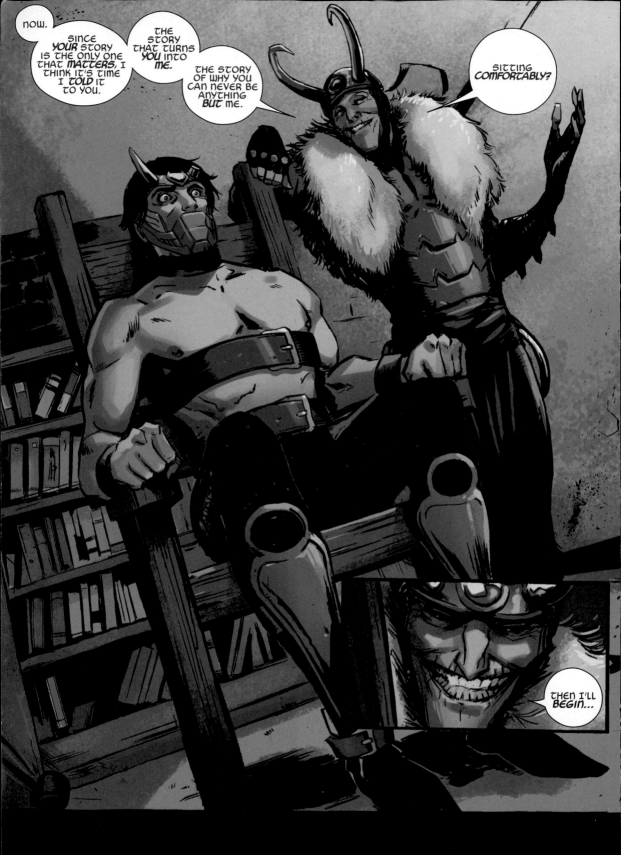

NEXT: EVERYTHING DIES.

COVER SKETCHES
by Lee Garbett

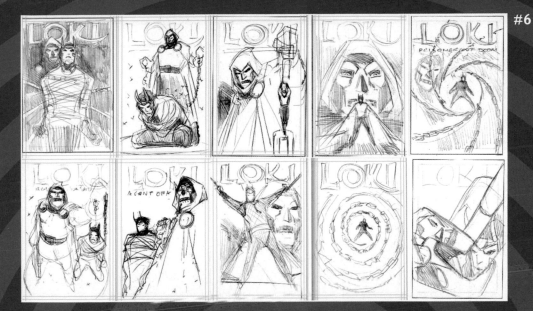

#6

#7

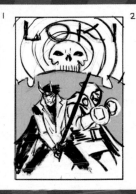

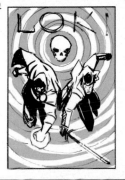

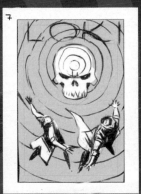

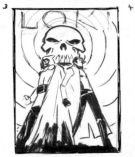

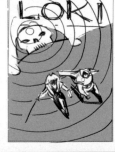

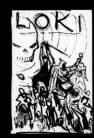

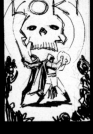

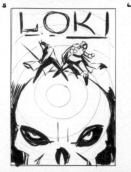

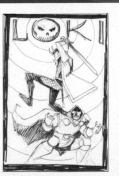

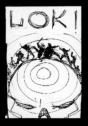

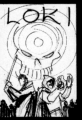

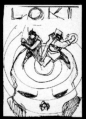

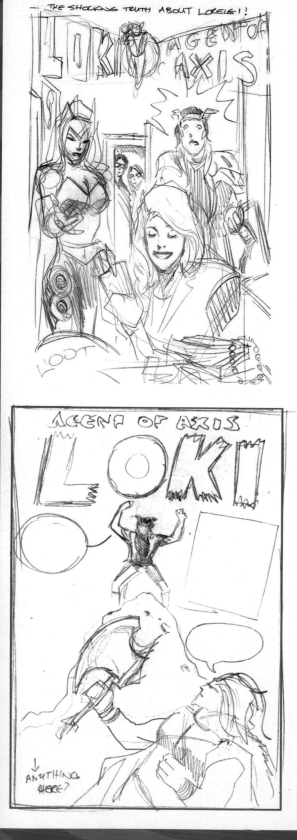

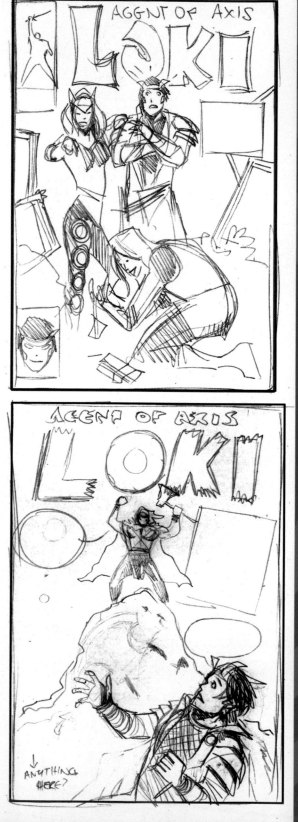

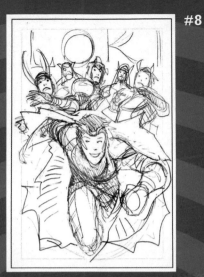

#8

#10

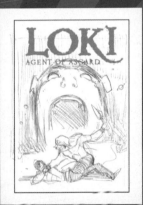

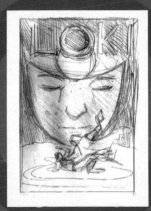

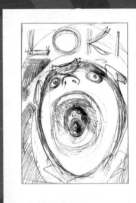

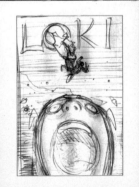

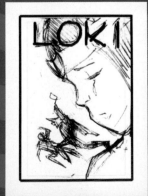

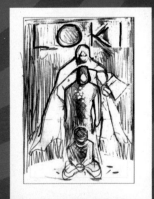

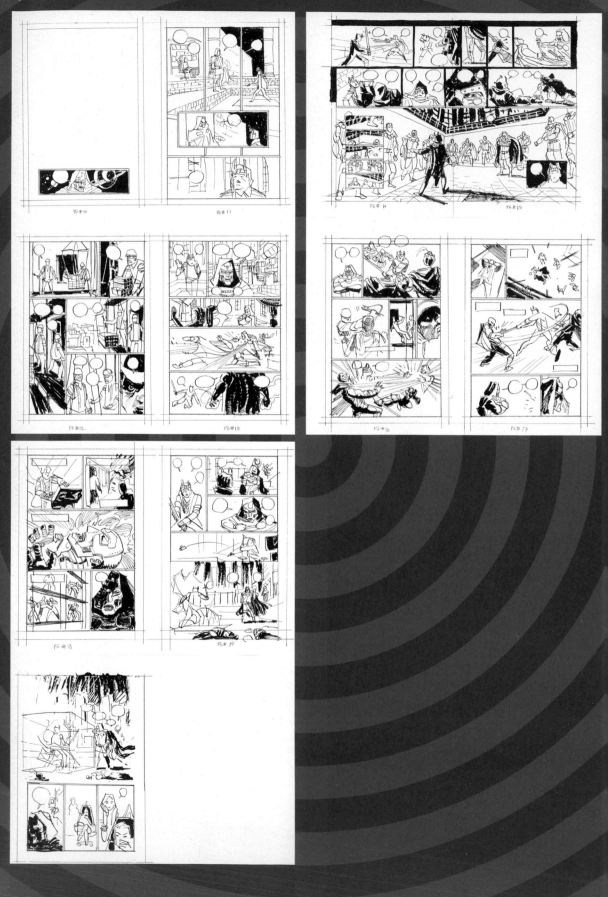

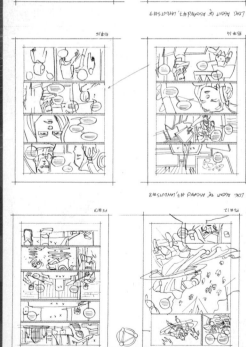
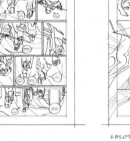
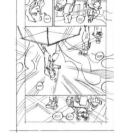
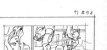
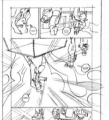
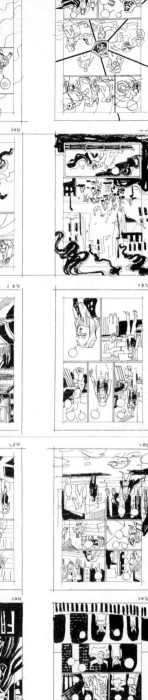
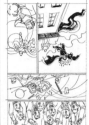
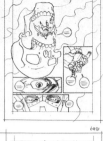
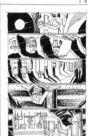
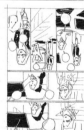
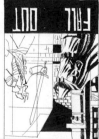
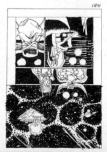
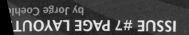

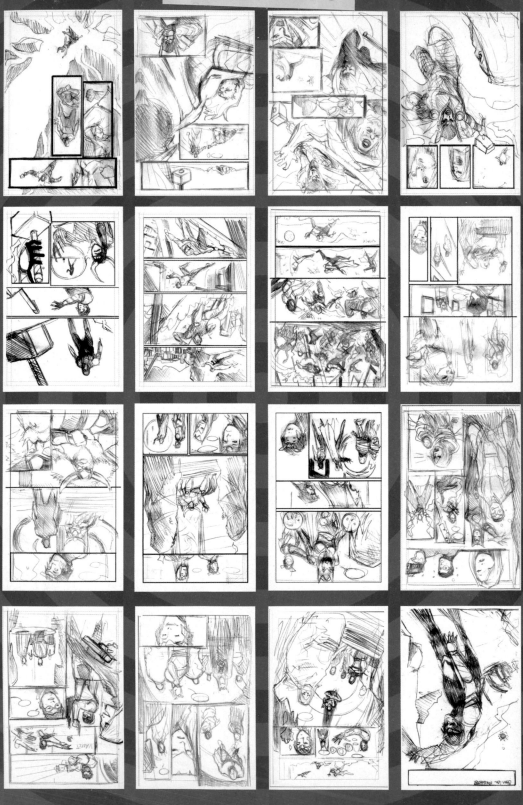